Vitality Now! A Complete Anti-aging Guide to Enhance Your Health and Vitality

Vitality Now! A Complete Anti-aging Guide to Enhance Your Health and Vitality

Karen Sun, M.D.

PUBLISHER'S NOTE
AN IMPORTANT CAUTION TO OUR READERS:

ISBN 978-1-300-81075-9

Cover design: Published by: Sunshine Publications
4 Hughes, Suite 150
Irvine, CA 92618

Dedication

This book is dedicated to all the teachers I encountered in my life and all my patients who I learned from their experience about healthy aging, disease prevention, and hormone balance.

Acknowledgements

I wish to thank my editors, researchers and fact checkers, Sebastien Cervantes and Roger Cervantes for their dedication, efforts and support. I wish to extend my heartfelt thanks to Rose Riojas, my business consultant, for her strategic advice, counsel and unwavering support. I want to thank my medical office manager, Crystal Soto, who handles all the daily and challenging tasks with a Zen-like attitude. I also wish to deeply thank my son, Michael, for his patience, love and support throughout this process.

Table of Contents

Introduction.. xvii

       My Story.. xviii

       My Observations..xxi

       My Theory... xxii

Part I: Understanding the Disease Process and Aging.............1

Chapter 1:   How Diseases Start......................................3

       Root Causes of Diseases..4

       Four Factors that Influence Health.........................5

       Activating Your Healing Systems..........................6

Chapter 2:   Theories of Aging...7

       Gene Control Theory and Telomeres.....................7

       Neuroendocrine Theory...8

       Free Radicals and Oxidative Stress Theory...........9

       Other Theories...10

       Summary...12

Part II: Hormone Balance...13

Chapter 3:   Menopause and Bio-identical Hormone
       Replacement Therapy...15

       What Are Sex Hormones?......................................16

       What Are the Functions of Sex Hormones?.........18

       Bio-identical versus Synthetic Hormones.............20

       Why Do We Need Hormone Replacement
       Therapy?...22

       Breast Cancer and Hormone Replacement
       Therapy (HRT)..23

Hormone Replacement Therapy – Routes of Delivery 27

Rules of Hormone Replacement 30

Chapter 4: Subcutaneous Bio-identical Hormone Pellet Implants 33

The Ultimate Hormone Replacement Therapy 33

Advantages of Pellet Therapy Demonstrated in Studies 33

Implant Procedure 35

Biological Action of Implants 36

Frequently Asked Questions 36

Indications for Pellet Therapy 38

Best Candidates for Pellet Therapy 49

Breast Cancer and Hormone Therapy 55

Breast Cancer Prevention 57

HRT and Menopausal Women 59

Laboratory Testing for Hormones 59

Side Effects of Pellets Therapy 61

Contraindications for Pellet Therapy 62

Self-assessment for Estrogen Dominance and PMS 62

Self-assessment for Testosterone Deficiency 63

Points to Remember 64

Chapter 5: Male Testosterone Deficiency 65

Symptoms of Andropause and Testosterone Deficiency 67

Diagnosis of Testosterone Deficiency 67

Common Reasons for Testosterone-estrogen Imbalance 68

Testosterone and the Prostate Gland 68

Testosterone and Depression 69

Testosterone and the Cardiovascular System 70

Testosterone and Insulin — Diabetes 71

Testosterone and Alzheimer's Disease 73

Testosterone and Osteoporosis 74

Is Testosterone Replacement Therapy the
Answer for Aging Men? 74

Testosterone — Routes of Delivery 75

Rules of Testosterone Replacement......................76

Indications for Testosterone Replacement............77

Side Effects of Testosterone Replacement 77

Contraindications for Testosterone
Replacement 77

Points to Remember..78

Chapter 6: Adrenal Fatigue — The Stress Epidemic 79

Stress Factors...79

Adrenal Hormones and Their Actions..................80

Stages of Stress and Adrenal Fatigue 80

Symptoms of Adrenal Exhaustion........................83

Diagnosis and Tests for Adrenal Fatigue.............83

Treatment of Adrenal Fatigue..............................84

Take Control of Your Diet — The Adrenal
Recovery Diet...86

Reduce Your Stress...86

Supplements for Recovery from Adrenal
Fatigue 88

Points to Remember..91

Chapter 7: Hypothyroidism — The Hidden Epidemic...........93

Hypothyroidism 94

Functions of Thyroid Hormones..........................95

Causes of Hypothyroidism 96

Symptoms of Hyperthyroidism.............................98

Signs of Hypothyroidism.....................................99

Diseases Frequently Associated with
Hypothyroidism..99

Diagnosis of Hypothyroidism 99

Treating Hypothyroidism 101

Self-assessment for Hypothyroidism 103

Points to Remember 104

Chapter 8:　Regenerative Medicine 105

Human Growth Hormone and Stem Cell
Treatment 105

Human Growth Hormone 105

Stem Cell Treatment 107

Part III: The Body, Mind, and Spirit Connection 111

Chapter 9:　Nutrition — You Are What You Eat 113

Breakdown on Nutrients 114

Anti-inflammation Diet 126

Weight Loss Diet 127

Healthy Aging Diet 129

Alkaline Diet 129

Points to Remember 130

Chapter 10:　Intestinal Health — Our First Line of Defense... 133

The GI Tract 133

Components of the GI Tract 133

Beneficial Bacteria 136

GERD 136

Leaky Gut Syndrome and Food 137

Diagnosis of Leaky Gut Syndrome 141

Treatment of Leaky Gut Syndrome 142

Candida 145

Self-assessment for Leaky Gut 146

Interpreting the Results 147

Summary 148

Chapter 11:　Our Toxic World — The Silent Killer 149

Types of Toxins 153

Sources of Chemicals in the Environment..........163

Toxin Avoidance — How to Avoid Exposure
to Toxins..164

How the Body Detoxifies....................................165

Electromagnetic Frequency (EMF)
Contamination..174

Multiple Chemical Sensitivities..........................176

Chapter 12:   How to Look 10 Years Younger — Beauty Is Not
Just Skin Deep..179

The Skin..179

Epidermis, Outer Layer.......................................180

Dermis: The Middle Layer...................................181

Subcutaneous: The Inner Layer...........................181

Principles of Keeping Your Skin Youthful.........182

Treatment for Pigmented Skin Blotches and
Sun Spots...183

Laser and IPL...184

Home Skin Care...185

Chapter 13:   Our Mind — You Are What You Think.............187

The Mind — Body Connection............................187

Neurotransmitters and the Neuroendocrine
Communication System..190

Brain Health and Hormones................................192

How to Improve Brain Health.............................194

The Conscious, Subconscious, and
Unconscious Mind...195

Meditation..196

Steps for Creative Visualization, Guided
Imaginary and Positive Affirmations:.................196

Self-esteem..198

Chapter 14:   Spirit — Your True Power...............................201

Anatomy of the spirit..201

Training for Positive Thoughts and Emotions 203

Our Belief System — Philosophy Toward Life .. 204

Part IV: Healthy Aging Program 209

Chapter 15:   Prevention of Disease... 211

Cardiovascular Disease — Hypertension,
Heart Attack, and Stroke 211

Diagnostic Tests for Screening Cardiovascular
Diseases.. 213

Prevention of Cardiovascular Disease 215

Balance Your Hormones..................................... 216

Cancer 217

Diagnostic Testing for Early Cancer Detection .. 217

Cancer Prevention 220

Metabolic Syndrome — Insulin Resistance,
Obesity, and Diabetes 223

Laboratory Testing... 224

Prevention and Treatment of Metabolic
Syndrome 225

Premature Brain Aging, Memory Loss,
Neurodegenerative Disease, Impaired 226

Cognition, and Dementia 226

Prevention of Neurodegenerative Diseases........ 227

Osteoporosis and Osteopenia 229

Chapter 16:   8 Weeks to Vitality 233

Week 1 — Health Assessment............................ 233

Week 2 — Hormone Balance 237

Week 3 — Make Sleep a Priority, Check Your
Stress Inventory, and Take Control.................... 237

Week 4 — Better Nutrition and Healthy Diet..... 242

Week 5 — Adding Exercise to Your Daily
Routine 250

Week 6 — Toxin Avoidance, Detoxification,
and Reevaluation.. 252

Week 7 — Unleash Your Subconscious Power ..253

Daily Planning 254

Week 8 — Putting It All Together 254

Summary...256

Recommended Reading....................................257

References...261

Index 271

Introduction

Are you a middle-aged woman suffering from hot flashes, insomnia, moodiness, and weight gain? Are you a middle-aged man suffering from declining energy, memory, and libido? Are you curious about the pros and cons of hormone replacement therapy, and what form is the safest and most effective? Are you aware of the toxins in our environment and the ways to help your body detoxify?

Do you want to reduce your stress levels, and experience more peace and joy in your life? Do you want to know how to eat in order to reduce inflammation, indigestion, and lose weight? Do you want to prevent heart disease, stroke, cancer, and Alzheimer's disease? Do you want to slow the aging process down and regain the vitality you once had?

If you answered "yes" to any of the questions above, this book is for you, as it has been written for people who want to take charge of their health and healing. Knowledge is power, and the more you know about your body and the many factors that influence your health and well-being, the more empowered you will be to make informed decisions that will improve the quality of your life.

The quest to achieve a true and lasting healing of the body and to balance those needs with those of the mind and spirit is a goal that many share, and one that I have pursued throughout my professional career. The search has been exhaustive, with gains and setbacks along the way. What I have discovered are the keys to balancing the fundamental cornerstones of our physical, mental, and emotional health, well into mature adulthood. This journey has enabled thousands of patients to regain their vitality and enjoy healthy and active lives at any age. In this book I would like to share these discoveries with you.

My Story

Throughout my life, I have always been accustomed to fast paced living. Like most of the women I see in my practice, I have to juggle multiple roles: long hours of work, worrying about the health of my patients, and trying to be a good mother at the same time. The challenges have been never ending. Like most women, I have been the last person I have time for.

My health was not great in my younger years. I developed scoliosis early in life and suffered through many years of neck and back pain. My stomach became extremely sensitive, and I had bad reactions to many types of foods with abdominal pain and bloating. My energy fluctuated throughout the day, even after a full night's rest. I also experienced heavy menstrual bleeding and cramps. Yet, despite the clear warning signs that my body was sending, I continued to press on, convinced that the rewards of a fast-paced lifestyle were more than worth the effort.

By the time I entered menopause in my early fifties, things had changed. I had hot flashes that awakened me and poor sleep that lead to a decline in memory and energy. Handling daily tasks became more difficult. My skin became dryer. I had more aches and pains and nothing seemed to interest me. I became frustrated, to say the least. My OB/GYN suggested antidepressants for the hot flashes and to help improve my sleep. Being an internist, I knew better than to risk the potential side effects of these drugs. I did not like the idea of taking birth control pills or oral estrogen, since their side effects are well documented. My desire to avoid the use of heavy-duty drugs led me to try a more benign approach which included natural hormones like progesterone creams and estradiol patches, knowing they would attempt to mimic the hormones my body once produced. Due to my hectic schedule, however, I would often forget to reapply the creams or replace the patches, only to wake up with night sweats the next night. Plus, I was still tired throughout the day and not feeling well overall.

The answer came one day during a routine consultation when one of my patients introduced me to a book about implanted bio-identical hormone pellet therapy. I initially reacted with skepticism. Many questions came to mind, such as: What is this? Why have I not heard about this? Is it dangerous? I had many reservations about the book. Yet by this time the undesirable symptoms associated with my transition into menopause, coupled with the aches and pains accumulated from my overworked lifestyle, had become a constant ordeal. My experience with hormone creams and patches had already opened my eyes to the possibilities of hormone therapy, so I set aside my doubts and read the book. Interestingly, I found that the information it contained made a great deal of sense and is based on solid medical research.

Encouraged by this, I made the decision to be trained to do this procedure. Right after the training, I treated a few of my patients who were not responding to hormone creams and patches with severe menopausal symptoms with the pellets. The results were immediate and startling. Every one of these patients experienced a dramatic improvement! So, I decided to begin treatment with bio-identical hormone pellets on myself. It turned out to be one of the best decisions I have ever made. My symptoms disappeared! As a matter of fact, the third morning after the pellet implant I slept like a baby, arose early in the morning refreshed, and went for a vigorous jog. I felt energetic and happy and healthy for the first time in a long time

I started introducing the pellets to some of my patients who had been using hormone creams with questionable results. Their improvement was immediate and noticeable as well. Symptoms that responded only mildly to hormone creams disappeared completely once the pellets were implanted. As a result of the wonderful improvement in my patient's health, the news began to spread. As everyone knows, a good secret can be hard to keep, especially when the benefits are so readily apparent both inside and out, as they clearly are with bio-identical hormone therapy. A steady stream of patient referrals began to inundate my appointment lists. Many of these new patients had to drive hours to get to my practice, and quite a few traveled from out of state. Many patients were desperate to find relief after having exhausted just about every other means of conventional and alternative treatments and had heard of my success treating patients with bio-identical hormone pellet therapy. So beneficial were these powerful little pellets, and so rapid was the spread of their praise, that within a span of six years my practice grew to more than 3,000 patients who were benefiting from bio-identical hormone pellet therapy; a powerful testimony to its effectiveness.

Gradually, men began showing up in my office. Usually their wive's or girlfriend's had received treatment from me first. After witnessing the dramatic change their partner had experienced, particularly with their improved libido, these men became eager to try this treatment for themselves. It is no longer a secret that men can benefit from pellet therapy, especially professional men with stressful jobs, who, upon reaching middle-age, find themselves becoming more irritable and short tempered and feel they are losing energy, mental sharpness, and vitality. Many of the men who come to see me have heard of testosterone shots, but they are unaware of the many advantages in safety and efficacy which bio-identical testosterone pellets offer. Once they experience the remarkable benefits of treatment, most men are quick to embrace this approach as well.

There is no doubt pellet therapy can be a powerful and life-altering experience for many people. In my quest to fulfill my patients' desires for optimal health, I came to realize that hormones are only one part of the solution. I continued my study and research, and attended seminars offered by organizations such as The American College of Advanced Medicine (ACAM) and The Institute of Functional medicine (IFM). From those seminars, I learned how to treat the root causes of disease, not just the symptoms. I also learned how to combine conventional treatment methods with alternative approaches to produce therapies that work. Although I have been board certified in internal medicine for over twenty-five years, in 2010 I decided to expand my medical awareness and became board certified in integrative and holistic medicine. The path to achieve healthy aging led me to discover I had multiple internal ailments that are quite common among women today. I had food allergies due to mercury and candida, and I also had adrenal fatigue due to chronic stress. To cure myself of these ailments I needed to change my eating patterns, take supplements, add daily exercise, and train my mind and thoughts.

I want the reader to know I recently felt the need to personally explore stem cell treatments for my own medical well-being. I traveled to a medical clinic in China and feel strongly about the positive results I have achieved from this treatment. I encourage the reader to examine and consider all the available medical alternatives and question their applicability to your concerns with your physician.

During the course of my practice in medicine, I also came to realize treating the body is not enough. The body also houses our mind and spirit. Unless the mind and spirit are at ease, the body will become diseased. Many of my patients are no different than your friends, neighbors, and relatives. Modern living has given us anxiety and stress related disorders which we all suffer from sometime. However, these problems will sometimes force us to stop and examine our lives, and by doing this, we realize we need to make changes. Thus, we should, at times, be grateful this has happened, for it will force us to focus on the things in our lives which are genuinely important. Love is what is truly important, along with forgiveness and living in the present. We all have important missions to fulfill in our lives, and I believe we are here to learn lessons, enjoy life, and help other people as much as we can.

My Observations

Official statistics estimate the majority of women today suffer from a variety of unpleasant conditions during their menopausal years. While a small portion of women are able to make the transition through menopause with little to no difficulty, a roughly equal to greater number remain on the opposite end of the spectrum, suffering intensely from a variety of uncomfortable, and in many cases, debilitating health issues that dramatically affect their quality of life.

It has been my observation that most patients suffering from severe menopausal symptoms also have adrenal fatigue. This condition occurs when the adrenal glands function below their optimal levels and is usually caused by chronic stress. Before menopause, the adrenal glands contribute approximately 30 percent of the sex hormone production and more than 70 percent after menopause. When the adrenal glands become burned out, they are not able to produce the sex hormones a woman's body requires after menopause. I fit into this category as an overworked career woman. Patients with mild cases of adrenal fatigue respond wonderfully to pellet therapy, as it helps them to sleep better and increases their energy level. Patients in moderate to severe stages of adrenal fatigue need additional treatment, such as adrenal support products and vitamin supplements. Most importantly, however, they need to incorporate major lifestyle changes to reduce the stressors in their lives.

The thyroid is another hormone that plays a vital role in energy production. I have seen many patients with thyroid function tests in the lower range of normal that have all the symptoms of hypothyroidism. These people gain weight easily and have a hard time losing weight. This type of subclinical (undiagnosed) hypothyroidism is very common, especially in menopausal women, and a low dosage of thyroid medication helps provide health improvement.

I have also observed that certain patients have adverse responses to pellet therapy. In these cases, it is likely that their hormone receptors are altered, due to the effects of the accumulation of toxins in their bodies. Usually, they also suffer from other problems such as multiple chemical sensitivities, leaky gut syndrome, autoimmune diseases, or heavy metals such as mercury toxicity. This group of patients is more difficult to treat. Often, a detoxification program is a necessary first step in treatment. Also, due to their increased sensitivity their pellet dosages need to be carefully adjusted.

My Theory

Women are much more stressed now, due to juggling family lives and careers, not to mention taking care of everyone else's needs before their own. By the time menopause arrives, the adrenal glands are burned out when the ovaries have quit working. The adrenal glands are supposed to take over the production of sex hormones in women after menopause. But, due to adrenal fatigue, an increasing number of women are experiencing very uncomfortable and sometimes debilitating menopausal symptoms.

Men, on the other hand, are not much better off. Chronic stress also causes adrenal fatigue, which reduces testosterone production from the adrenal glands. Andropause, the term coined to describe male menopause, develops more gradually but earlier, with its own debilitating symptoms like low libido, fatigue, weight gain, mental fog, and cardiovascular diseases.

Stress management has become "Survival 101." Without changing our thoughts and value systems, we will not be able to gain control over the continual firing line of stressors we are exposed to in today's world. As we grow older, stress coping skills such as meditation, creative visualization, and relaxation exercises are important survival tools.

We also live in a very toxic world, tremendously more so than previous generations. By the time we reach middle-age, we have accumulated enough toxins in our body to seriously interrupt our hormone systems. The damage is more pervasive as the body's toxic load interferes with our brain functions and causes inflammation in the body that can lead to neurodegenerative diseases, cardiovascular diseases, and cancer. Because of each person's genetics are unique, the body's detoxification capacities differ. This is why some people, but not all, suffer from diseases like chronic fatigue syndrome, fibromyalgia, breast cancer, prostate cancer, and multiple chemical sensitivities. If we do not pay attention to the toxins in and around us, we run the risk of becoming victims of these diseases sooner or later.

Hormone balance is the first essential step to regain the vitality we once had and slow down the aging process, maintaining a better digestion and intestinal system, stress management and detoxification are the next steps, which involve lifestyle modification, developing stress coping skills, daily exercise routine, along with optimal nutrition and taking supplements that help the body detoxify. The last, and most important, step is achieving emotional and spiritual health.

It is my sincere hope that the information contained in this book helps you prevent disease, achieve optimal health, and defy aging, while experiencing peak physical vitality, mental clarity, and emotional well-being throughout your lifetime.

To your health!

Defy Aging

Hormone Balance and Beyond

Part I: Understanding the Disease Process and Aging

Chapter 1

How Diseases Start

Modern medicine has done great things to improve the quality of our lives. Over the course of the last century, its ability to understand disease has made incredible progress. Significant advances in key areas of medical research and technology have enabled physicians to employ increasingly sophisticated techniques in the treatment of illnesses. For example, impressive innovations in the field of diagnostic technology including imaging methods like computed tomography (CT) and magnetic resonance imaging (MRI) allow physicians to accurately and rapidly diagnose diseases in patients and help spot potential problems before they occur. Major advances in surgery and medications have been made for treating cancer, heart disease, and other acute and chronic diseases.

Modern medicine also has major shortcomings. It focuses more on treating diseases rather than preventing them from occurring in the first place. With modern medicine's emphasis on medication or surgery as its main tools, it is much better suited to treat acute illnesses, rather than chronic conditions. Indeed, there are times when people need antibiotics to knock out infections or pain killers to alleviate headaches. But for chronic illnesses such as hypertension, diabetes or arthritis, treatment by medication alone solves only part of the problem. Consideration must also be given to proper nutrition and necessary lifestyle practices, such as maintaining proper weight, getting regular exercise, managing stress, and avoiding tobacco as well as excessive use of alcohol.

Another concern about modern medicine is that it divides diseases into separate systems instead of viewing the body's systems as closely interrelated. Specialists and sub-specialists for everything worsen this fragmented perspective. While focusing on a single system has helped doctors to better understand the disease process within each system of the body, this narrow view often ignores the fact that a symptom can have complex causative factors involving multiple body systems. A headache, for example, can be brought on by emotional issues, food sensitivities, hypertension, hormonal imbalance, recurring stress, allergies, or several of these factors combined. So, if a doctor were to treat a patient complaining of a headache with pain medication, the symptoms might well subside for the time being, but the underlying or root cause of the headache will not have been addressed. As a result, the headaches might continue to come back and neither patient nor physician will be aware of the deeper, persistent problems at work. Furthermore, the long-term use of pain medication carries with it the potential for dangerous side effects such as stomach ulcers, kidney or liver damage, and even addiction, all of which contribute to more health problems.

Symptoms are like the leaves on a tree. If you trim the leaves but leave the roots intact, the leaves are guaranteed to return. It is important to look for and treat the root causes of disease, so that patients can achieve a deep and truly effective healing: one that helps to ensure a lasting return to good health.

Root Causes of Diseases

We all inherit different sets of genes from our parents, which can make us prone to certain illnesses. This does not necessarily mean we will get these diseases. A lifestyle burdened by unhealthy habits, however, can make these diseases much more likely to affect us. If adult onset (Type II) diabetes runs in your family, and if you live a sedentary lifestyle that includes poor diet and lack of exercise, then the likelihood you will develop diabetes dramatically increases. But, if you watch your diet, exercise regularly, maintain proper weight, and manage stressors well, then your likelihood of developing diabetes is greatly reduced.

Lifestyle is a major factor that has the power to aggravate or prevent many diseases. This is true not only for genetically inherited diseases but for many other diseases as well.

Four Factors that Influence Health

The following four factors play a major role in determining an individual's overall health and well-being. Maintaining a healthy balance between these factors is especially important for individuals whose bodies have begun to curtail or cease production of the vital hormones that allow us to cope with stressors and imbalances in our lifestyles.

1. Nutrition and intact gut: We are what we eat. Eating a balanced diet helps to build a strong body. The GI (gastrointestinal) tract plays an important role in our health, as its functions are digestion, absorption of nutrients, waste elimination, and detoxification. It also serves as a first line of defense to prevent toxins, bacteria, or large food molecules from entering our bodies.

2. Mental processes: We are what we think. The mind is the arbiter of our thoughts and emotions. Positive thoughts lead to a mental state where feelings of peace, calm, and happiness flow naturally and lead to optimal function of the body. A consistently negative outlook on life can make one far more vulnerable to anxiety, depression, worry, anger, and fear, thus triggering the body's stress response.

3. Toxins: We live in a world full of toxins. Our body also produces free radicals through chemical reactions that are continually occurring. If we are exposed to more toxins than our body's detoxification system can handle, or more free radicals than our antioxidants can neutralize, then toxins start to accumulate, leading to inflammation and aging. Toxins cause inflammation, which contributes to degenerative diseases like arthritis, atherosclerosis, or Alzheimer's disease. Toxins also cause DNA mutations that lead to cancer. Additionally, toxins weaken our immune system, which leads to allergies, infections, and autoimmune diseases.

4. Hormones: Our body's hormones are the chemical messengers which govern how cells, tissues, and organs communicate with each other. There are many different kinds of hormones that are typically categorized as either

major or minor, depending upon the role they play and the amount of influence they exert upon our body's functions. Certain major hormones such as thyroid and adrenal hormones are so critical to our health that without them we run the risk of disease and death. Without minor hormones like estrogen and testosterone, our body's ability to function optimally is critically impaired.

If our hormones are in plentiful supply, balanced, and working together then our body will have the tools it needs to function optimally. We will look our best, feel our best, and enjoy the benefits of renewed energy and vitality as the aging process dramatically slows down.

In addition to exerting a fundamental influence on our health, all four of these factors are closely interrelated. If you suffer from hormonal imbalance, for instance, you may feel tired, depressed, moody, or anxious. If you are stressed, you may not eat the best foods, exercise properly, or sleep well. If you are exposed to certain toxins that disrupt your thyroid hormones, you will gain weight and feel sluggish, even if you eat well and exercise regularly.

Activating Your Healing Systems

Having a healthy body is important, but the extent in which we can fully embrace optimum health is largely determined by our mental and emotional state as well. A healthy body depends on an active, alert mind, which, in turn, draws support from our balanced emotions and strength of spirit. This vital balance of mind, body, and spirit is the cornerstone of our health and well-being. In order to get well and stay well, we need to manage all the root factors of disease in order to promote our own internal healing systems.

The answer to the wide array of issues facing our health in the world today lies in a multifaceted approach that takes each aspect of our individuality into account. If we improve our nutritional habits, make exercise a priority, foster emotional wellbeing, reduce the stressors in our lives, balance our hormones, maintain proper weight, avoid tobacco and excessive alcohol, and use supplements to aid in the prevention of disease, we will have taken crucial and empowering steps toward the goal of living long, healthy, and happy lives.

Chapter 2

Theories of Aging

A few years ago I attended my forty-year high school reunion. Since I had gone to an all-girls' school, I saw a room full of middle-aged women. They had familiar faces and voices, yet were very different from what I remembered during our teenage years. Some had gained a lot of weight, and others had gray hair. But even those who had not gained weight or grayed still had different faces, due to sagging skin that had fine wrinkles or lost its elasticity. I felt that I was in a time machine tunnel that had moved way too fast!

While aging is an inevitable fact of life, there are many things we can do to slow the process down. Before we discuss these approaches, let us take a moment to go behind the scenes of the aging process and examine its primary causes. Along with the many advances in the study of medicine today, several promising theories have come that help to explain the fundamental causes of aging.

Gene Control Theory and Telomeres

Each time a cell in the body duplicates, it creates entirely new structures of DNA called chromosomes. Telomeres (derived from the Greek sub-specialists, or end, and meres, or part) are small fragments of DNA that form the protective ends of chromosomes. The telomeres protect a cell's chromosomes from fusing with each other or rearranging. Each time the chromosomes duplicate, the telomeres get a little shorter, and after their structures shrink to a certain size, cell division stops. At this point, no additional new cells can be made

One abnormality of this cell duplication process is a genetic disorder called progeria, an accelerated aging disease. Progeria is an extremely rare condition. An individual affected by progeria looks like a miniature elderly person and they typically do not live past ten years of age. Children afflicted with this condition develop the diseases associated with aging, such as arthritis, osteoporosis, and heart attacks.

Diseases like progeria have helped to increase attention on the issues of aging and longevity and their link to our genes. Studies have observed that certain species of animals have programmed life spans. For human beings, the genetic potential for longevity has been estimated at about 120 years. Most people, however, never meet this potential due to premature aging, or because they are genetically susceptible to certain diseases.

Genetic engineering has been a controversial subject for many years. Research in genetic engineering has led to improvements in agricultural crop technology, and the manufacturing of synthetic human insulin through the use of modified bacteria.

Will advances in gene therapy and genetic engineering someday provide the keys to unlocking our vast lifespan? Possibly, but it is important to remember that the human body is a complex organism. Many questions concerning genes and their effect on the human body still remain unanswered. Although research continues to make strides forward, it must be tempered by respect for what "Mother Nature" has already accomplished and the knowledge that the artificial manipulation of genes has the potential to backfire.

Neuroendocrine Theory

The Neuroendocrine Theory was first proposed in 1954 by the well-known Russian gerontologist, Vladimir Dilman. Professor Dilman believed the cause of aging could be traced directly to the loss of sensitivity that occurred in the hypothalamus, a walnut sized gland located in the brain. A large amount of hormones are needed to repair and regulate our body's functions and are regulated by the hypothalamus. The hypothalamus controls high level chain reactions which instruct organs and glands like the pituitary, pineal, and thymus glands to release hormones to our body as needed.

The pituitary gland secretes HGH (human growth hormone) to regulate growth, TSH (thyroid-stimulating hormone) to regulate thyroid hormones, ACTH (adrenocorticotropic hormone) to regulate the adrenal glands, and FSH (follicle- stimulating hormone) and LH (luteinizing hormone) to regulate estrogen, testosterone, and progesterone.

The pineal gland, also located in the brain, secretes melatonin, which regulates sleep patterns. In the chest, just behind the breast bone, is the thymus gland, which stimulates certain infection-fighting cells to boost the immune system.

As we age, our hormone levels decline. This translates to the body's reduced ability to regulate and repair itself. Much like an old car that requires regular tune-ups and maintenance, the body depends upon optimal hormone levels to repair damaged tissue so the body can function at its best. Without such care to the car, it runs the risk of breaking down very quickly. If done correctly, replacing the declining hormones helps to slow down or even reverse the aging process in our bodies.

Free Radicals and Oxidative Stress Theory

The Free Radical and Oxidative Stress Theory was developed by Dr. Denham Harman and introduced during the 1950s. Since then it has become widely regarded as one of the most popular and influential theories on the aging process, helping to spark strong public interest in the concepts of anti-aging, age-related diseases, and antioxidant supplementation. Today, terms like "free radicals" and "antioxidants" are a part of our common vocabulary, but in order to go beyond the buzz words and learn more about this concept we need to explore some of the lesser known functions of the body, beginning with electrons.

Electrons are required to produce electricity. The body also has an electrical system which utilizes electrons to perform its many vital functions, such as contraction of the heart and skeletal muscles, as well as to ensure that each of the body's organs and tissues work properly.

A car burns gasoline to produce energy, creating toxic exhaust as a by- product. The body behaves in much the same way, burning sugar to produce energy in a process called oxidation. One of the main side effects of oxidation is the production of extra electrons, called free radicals, which are the body's own toxic exhaust. Unfortunately, extra free radicals circulating in the body attack and interfere with the functions of our cells. This free radical damage is called oxidative stress, which starts as soon as we are born. When we are young, the body has high levels of hormones to combat this oxidative stress and reduce the inflammation caused by the free radicals. As we grow older, our dropping hormone levels are not able to protect us from the damage of free radicals to our tissues, leading to inflammation, tissue destruction, and aging.

Environmental toxins can also pose a hazardous threat; acting either like free radicals in the body or by directly damaging our cells, or by a combination of both negative effects. As we age, we are exposed to more toxins. Our environment, compared to the past, has more chemicals which infiltrate our water systems, foods, consumer products, and the air. Many of these chemicals are not biodegradable, meaning they will continue to persist in our environment for generations to come. The long- term impact these new toxins have on our planet and the human race has yet to be determined.

Substances which neutralize free radicals and prevent the harmful effects of oxidation are known as antioxidants. Eating fruits and vegetables supplies natural antioxidants to combat damage from free radicals. Other beneficial substances, called free radical scavengers, seek out free radicals and bind them before they attack body cells. Many vitamins and minerals are both antioxidants and free radical scavengers and also help the body's detoxification process. Accordingly, if we can reduce the damage generated by free radicals and oxidative stress, we can slow the aging process.

Other Theories

Mitochondrial Depletion

The energy producers for our body are tiny mitochondria found in each cell. When mitochondria quit working due to DNA damage, toxins, nutritional deficiency, or hormonal imbalance, we become very fatigued. Loss of mitochondrial energy production will lead to cell and tissue death. Many nutritional supplements such as alpha lipoic acid, CoQ 10 and magnesium can support mitochondria function.

Chronic Inflammation

Recent research has identified chronic inflammation as a common, underlying factor in several age related diseases like Alzheimer's disease, heart disease, diabetes and arthritis. Inflammation is our body's first line of defense against infection. When we are hurt or injured, immune cells respond quickly to prevent the spread of infection and repair damaged tissue. However, chronic inflammation, which can be caused by oxidative stress, chronic infection, accumulated toxins, or hormonal imbalance mistakenly signals our immune systems to continue this process, turning a healthy mechanism for healing into a continued assault upon otherwise healthy body structures. Left unchecked, this process can lead to a host of ill effects which help speed up the aging process.

Digestive Enzyme Deficiency

Digestive enzymes play a central role in our body's ability to break down and process the food we eat. Through the chemical reactions they create, our food is converted into the essential nutrients that our bodies require in order to build and repair cells, tissues, and organs. As we age, the number of digestive enzymes we are able to secrete declines, a process that eventually leads to inefficient digestion and absorption of nutrients. Without the ability to fully utilize vital nutrients, our body cannot function optimally, allowing the aging process to accelerate at a faster rate. Simply taking digestive enzyme with your meals and eating smaller meals will help the digestive process and, thus, your nutritional status.

Circulatory Deficiency

The circulatory system is our body's super highway. This amazing infrastructure composed of the heart, blood, and blood vessels connects all of the body's cells and is responsible for transporting nutrients, oxygen, and water throughout the body. A healthy, functioning circulatory system is critical to our body's ability to maintain optimum health. When the circulatory system's ability to deliver crucial nutrients is hampered, a number of problems can develop. Atherosclerosis, a hardening of the arteries, leads to poor circulation due to narrowing of the blood vessels. Reduced circulation to the capillaries in the eyes can lead to blindness, and reduced circulation to the brain can cause senility. Like an irrigation canal to crops, reduced circulation in our bodies leads to worn out and poorly performing organs.

Summary

Normal aging and pathological aging or premature aging are different. Normal aging is a process that occurs in every living organism. Our bodies are no exception to this rule, and normal age progression is recognized as a part of the cycle of life. However, pathological or premature aging is quite different. It is not a normal aging process and is brought on by diseases such as Alzheimer's, diabetes, heart disease, and strokes, conditions that are largely preventable by improving the health and quality of our lifestyles.

The causes of premature aging are quite similar to the root causes of diseases. Many of the causative factors involved in the disease process lie in the choices we make each day. Poor nutrition, obesity, lack of exercise, excessive tobacco and alcohol consumption, and over-reliance on medications contribute to a large portion of this process. The power to change begins with us, and we can make the decision to take positive steps toward better health today, by making simple adjustments to our daily habits and lifestyle choices.

Making the commitment to achieve emotional well-being and reduce the stress in our lives is critical as well. The time and effort we spend detoxifying our negative thoughts and minimizing stressors at work and home will pay lasting dividends. These self-empowering choices will help form the foundation of optimum health.

As medical research advances and gives us more options to use in our healing process, and as you and I choose to make positive changes, changes in our eating choices, eliminating toxins, improving our mental outlook, and physical wellbeing and, of course, balancing our hormones, we can immensely improve our quality of life. We now have the ability to slow down the aging process and return to you the youthful energy, vitality, and healthy outlook about the future we once had.

Part II: Hormone Balance

Chapter 3

Menopause and Bio-identical Hormone Replacement Therapy

Making the transition through menopause can be a turbulent and distressing time for women. The physical discomfort, emotional unrest, and lack of energy that accompany this midlife process can take a huge toll on women's vitality, usually when they need it the most.

Every day I see women in my office with similar stories. They have worked hard all of their lives either raising families, as business professionals, or both. Now they have reached menopause and without warning their lives have suddenly started to deteriorate. Hot flashes keep them awake at night and the interrupted sleep leads to fatigue. They gain weight, even with more exercise and less food. Their moods become crabby and irritable. They are unable to concentrate and have poor memories. They experience increasing vaginal dryness making intercourse painful, which often is enough to kill any libido that remains. Their skin becomes dry and itchy, wrinkles creep up on their face, their breasts sag, and more fat begins to accumulate around their abdominal area. They look in the mirror and are horrified at what they have become.

Some choose to suffer through these symptoms in silence without getting any type of hormone replacement treatment due to fear of breast cancer. Some try over-the-counter remedies such as Estroven, black cohosh, or progesterone cream. Some are treated with birth control pills, antidepressants, or sleeping pills. Some receive conventional hormone treatment with Premarin® and/or progestin. Others try bio-identical hormone treatment with hormone creams, patches, or gels.

The patients who come to see me often do so because the treatments they tried had little effect or bothersome side effects. They have heard from friends that the treatments I applied have changed their lives. Thanks to treatment with bio-identical hormone implanted pellets, their friends now sleep better without hot flashes or night sweats, their energy levels have soared, their moods are improved, and their libido has returned. It is easier for them to lose weight and, best of all, they feel young again. Their sense of well-being has returned and they no longer feel trapped in a menopausal state.

Naturally these women come with all sorts of questions. If this is such a wonderful treatment, why haven't their doctors told them about it? Is it safe? Will it cause breast cancer? How are the hormone pellets implanted under the skin? How long do they last? What types of side effects occur? These are good questions, and their answers will help you better understand this effective treatment for any menopausal symptoms you may be experiencing. Let us start by examining the basic physiology of hormones. This information will assist you in understanding the variety of treatment options available so you can make an informed decision when it comes to choosing the safest, most effective form of hormone replacement for your needs.

What Are Sex Hormones?

The sex hormones consist of three types: estrogens, progesterone, and testosterone. Both men and women have all three hormones, but estrogen is predominant in women and testosterone is predominant in men.

Sources of Sex Hormones

1. Ovaries: The ovaries are the body's primary source of estrogen and progesterone before menopause. There are three forms of estrogen in the human body: estrone (E1), estradiol (E2), and estriol (E3). As you can see from the figure below, they show only a slight difference in their molecular structures. However, these subtle differences lead to quite

important distinctions in the roles they perform. Before menopause, the ovaries mostly secrete estradiol, which accounts for the functions of estrogen we see in young women. Most of the positive effects of estrogen are due to estradiol. Estriol is produced in large amounts during pregnancy. It is a weak form of estrogen. Estrone and estradiol have to be metabolized into estriol before they can be excreted from the body. Our body needs estradiol to restore the normal physiology we had before menopause. Ovaries secrete progesterone only after ovulation, which happens at mid-cycle. After menopause the ovaries discontinue production of estrogen and progesterone, but continue to produce testosterone.

Natural Estrogens

Estradiol (E2)   Estrone (E1)   Estriol (E3)

2.   Adrenal glands: The adrenal glands produce DHEA, a hormone precursor which can convert into testosterone. They also produce pregnenolone, which can convert into cortisol, DHEA, progesterone, testosterone, and estrogen. The adrenal gland's contribution is critically important as they produce up to 30 percent of the sex hormone production in our younger years and after menopause become the major source of sex hormone production.

3.   Fat cells: Fat cells, especially those found in the abdominal area, can produce hormones. They secrete estrone. There is a theory that women gain fat after menopause in order to compensate for the demand of estrogen in the body. Researchers have found that the ratio of estrone to estradiol changes after menopause. Whereas higher levels of estradiol

are found in the body before menopause, that balance shifts to higher levels of estrone after menopause.

What Are the Functions of Sex Hormones?

Estrogen

1. Reproductive organs: The reproductive organs of the female body; the breasts, ovaries, vagina, and uterus all depend on the growth hormone estrogen. Without estrogen the body is negatively affected in numerous ways. For instance, breasts lose their volume and begin to sag. The lining of the uterus becomes atrophic (withered) and there are no more menstrual periods. Estradiol maintains the health of the cells of the vagina and urinary bladder, which reduces vaginal dryness and urinary problems like infections or incontinence.

2. Estradiol in the cardiovascular system. It dilates blood vessels, reducing blood pressure and limiting the formation of arteriosclerotic plaque on blood vessel walls. Loss of this estrogen is one of the reasons women tend to develop hypertension and cardiovascular disease after menopause. Insufficient estradiol also causes heart palpitations. Many women spend time and money having their hearts checked because of palpitations, only to discover that nothing is wrong and that the palpitations go away with adequate hormone replacement therapy.

3. Central nervous system: Estradiol increases blood flow to the brain protecting nerve cells and brain function. It has a deep impact on our central nervous system. By increasing neurotransmitters like acetylcholine and serotonin, estradiol helps with memory, relieves anxiety and depression, as well as promoting a normal sleep pattern. The sharp drop in estradiol makes it easy to see why many menopausal women complain of insomnia, anxiety, irritability, the inability to concentrate, and lack of mental alertness.

4. Skeletal system: Estradiol is also vital to the skeletal system. It reduces bone loss and helps our body make new bones. Lack of estrogen and other sex hormones in the long term

leads to brittle bones, a condition we call osteopenia, and as it progresses becomes osteoporosis. Estradiol also improves the connective tissues in the joints, thereby reducing the likelihood of the onset of degenerative arthritis.

5. Skin and hair: Estradiol helps to promote smoothness and elasticity of the skin, improves skin dryness, and prevents the loss of subcutaneous fat and collagen. Lack of it also leads to hair loss.

Progesterone

1. Balances estrogen: Progesterone helps to balance the effects of estrogen in the uterus and breast. Secreted by the ovaries after ovulation, it prevents overgrowth of the endometrium, the inner lining of the uterus. Menopausal women on HRT who still have a uterus need to take progesterone to prevent excessive buildup of the endometrium, which can lead to a heavy period and increase the possibility of getting endometrial cancer.

2. Protects the nervous system: Progesterone protects nerve cells and brain functions, and increases gamma-aminobutyric acid (GABA), a neurotransmitter that keeps us calmer and more relaxed. It also helps to restore normal sleep patterns.

3. Natural diuretic: Progesterone helps to prevent fluid retention by working as a natural diuretic.

4. Optimizes estrogen receptors: Lastly, progesterone helps estrogen receptors to function better.

Since nature designed progesterone to balance estrogen, much like the yin and yang, it is vital that levels of both hormones reach equilibrium to help maintain health. Estrogen dominance (excessive estrogen compared to progesterone), especially from environmental xenoestrogens, leads to fibrocystic breast disease, fibroid tumors, and even endometrial or breast cancer. When estrogen and progesterone are not balanced after ovulation, it leads to premenstrual tension or PMS, which includes such symptoms as heavy menstrual flow, fluid retention, moodiness, and migraine headaches.

Testosterone

Testosterone, considered by many to be a male sex hormone, is also important in women's health. Testosterone affects the body in many ways:

- Increases muscle mass
- Boosts libido
- Assists in bone building and helps prevent osteoporosis
- Plays a very important role in protecting the cardiovascular system
- Helps with mood and works as an antidepressant.
- It also helps keep the mind focused and sharp
- Promotes sensitivity to insulin and improves carbohydrate metabolism

Testosterone's role in men's health has been well researched. Yet, the role of testosterone in women's health has long been neglected. This is tragic since testosterone plays the same roles in both men and women. Women, however, only have about 10 percent of the amount of testosterone as men, which is why women in general are neither as aggressive nor muscular as men.

The body's production of testosterone drops by about half between the ages of thirty and fifty. Since the ovaries continue to produce testosterone after menopause, women do not experience the dramatic drop in testosterone that they do with estrogen and progesterone.

Bio-identical versus Synthetic Hormones

Bio-identical hormone replacement is clearly superior to conventional synthetic hormone replacement because of its nearly perfect similarity to the hormones the body naturally produces. That is why it is called bio-identical. Both bio-identical hormones and synthetic hormones are produced by pharmaceutical companies and are FDA (Food and Drug Administration) approved. Bio-identical hormones have molecular structures exactly the same as the body's hormones. Synthetic hormones mimic the body's hormones, but are not an exact match. When using hormone replacement, it makes sense to use bio-identical hormones, since they have virtually the same chemical structures as those made by the body. Examples of bio-identical estrogens that have been available to date are: Estrace®, Estradiol, Vivelle-Dot® patch, Climara® patch, bi-estrogen (bi-est) natural hormone cream or tri-estrogen (tri-est) natural hormone cream.

Typically, bio-identical hormones are derived from plant sources like yams or soy. Unfortunately, humans do not have the enzymes in their bodies to convert these substances into bio-identical hormones, so adding soy or yams to your diet will not raise your hormone levels. Rather, these hormones must be synthesized in such a way that they can be delivered safely in the body, such as with implanted pellets.

Hormones function by fitting into their own unique receptors which are on the membranes of the cells. Synthetic hormones that are not exactly identical to our own do not fit as well into the receptors and therefore may not be able to perform optimally. In addition, they can also produce side effects. Using synthetic hormones is comparable to opening a door with a copy of a key that is not identical to the original key; it may not open the door, or may open a wrong door.

The synthetic hormones Premarin® and Provera® are the most commonly used forms of hormone replacement therapy and the most studied to date. Premarin® is a brand name that stands for "pregnant mare's urine" and is produced by Wyeth Pharmaceuticals and has been in use since its introduction in the 1950s. This hormone medication is manufactured by keeping a mare in a constant state of pregnancy and inserting a catheter into the horse's urinary bladder to collect her urine. It is from this urine that "conjugated equine estrogen" is extracted, which is approximately 75 percent estrone (E1) and ten other forms of horse estrogens. The estrogen secreted by premenopausal women is primarily estradiol (E2), not estrone (E1). Replacing estrone instead of estradiol does not restore a woman's premenopausal physiology.

Provera® (or medroxyprogesterone) belongs to a class of drugs that are termed "progestins," which are synthetic progesterone. While it is supposed to perform the functions of progesterone, since it is not bio-identical, it can cause many negative side effects. Synthetic progestins were originally developed to be more potent and longer-lasting than natural equivalents. They are also patentable by the pharmaceutical companies who make them. It is important not to confuse progestins with progesterone since their actions are so different.

Why Do We Need Hormone Replacement Therapy?

The most common reason women seek hormone replacement therapy (HRT) is the many miserable symptoms which typically accompany menopause. Women suffer from hot flashes, which can be socially embarrassing during the day and usually wake them up in the middle of the night. This leads to poor quality of sleep and fatigue. They gain weight due to the slowdown in metabolism associated with diminished hormone levels. Additionally many suffer from moodiness, depression, anxiety, poor memory, lack of concentration and mental fog. At the same time, women suffer from lack of libido and painful intercourse, but are often too embarrassed to complain of these symptoms to their doctors.

The second reason women need HRT is to help prevent, as well as treat, diseases that are related to aging. Studies have shown HRT improves blood sugar control in patients with diabetes, lowers blood pressure in patients with hypertension, delays the onset and decreases the risk of Alzheimer's disease, reduces age related eye diseases such as macular degeneration, reduces the risk of colorectal cancer, and prevents osteoporosis and fracture.[1,2,3,4,5,6,7,8]

If you have a family history of diabetes, hypertension, dementia, macular degeneration, colorectal cancer, or osteoporosis, utilizing hormone replacement therapy is an important step you can take to prevent these deadly diseases.

The third reason to consider HRT is its ability to slow the aging process. Aging is significantly accelerated by hormone decline. By keeping hormones in the ranges we had during our thirties and forties, we can maintain our vitality, youthful appearance, and retard the aging process.

A century ago human life expectancy was fifty years; now it is about eighty years. It may become 100 years in the not-sodistant future. Thirty or more years of low hormone levels may well lead to a miserably poor quality of life. Imagine lying in a nursing home bed, wearing a diaper, and being confused most of the time. It is not a pretty picture.

Hormone replacement therapy relieves the suffering that comes with menopause. Adequate hormone therapy gives people the assurance they can enjoy life well into their golden years by preventing many of the diseases that accompany the aging process.

Breast Cancer and Hormone Replacement Therapy (HRT)

The most common reason women do not want HRT is due to the fear of breast cancer. Conventional thinking about hormones and breast cancer does not extend much beyond estrogen. As a matter of fact, there are many hormones that affect breast cancer in many different ways both positively and negatively. Those hormones include estrogens, progesterone, testosterone, DHEA, melatonin, oxytocin, insulin, T3 (thyroid hormone) and human growth hormone (HGH). It is important to pay attention to the levels of all these hormones when considering HRT.

Estrogen

- The Women's Health Initiative (WHI) study was designed to identify the potential benefits and risks of hormone replacement therapy. This study revealed that women who received estrogen only (Premarin®) did not have an increase in the occurrence of breast cancer. Only women who received Provera® in addition to Premarin® in the form of Prempro® had an increase in breast cancer risk from thirty per 10,000 women years to thirty-eight per 10,000 women years.[7,9]

- A Swiss HRT study of 23,000 women, most of them using estradiol rather than conjugated equine estrogens (Premarin®), showed an actual decrease in the death rate from breast cancer.[10]

- Two studies out of MD Anderson demonstrated that estrogen use in women with a prior history of breast cancer showed a lower recurrence rate compared to the control group.[11,12]

- A review article analyzed twenty-four studies on women with a prior history of breast cancer published from 1986 to 2001. The recurrence rate of breast cancer and mortality rate were compared in women who received HRT versus women who did not receive HRT after breast cancer treatment. The meta analysis(combining the data from all twenty-four studies and analyzing them together) showed that breast cancer survivors using HRT experienced a slightly reduced (8.2%) breast cancer recurrence rate, and an almost four times reduction in mortality rate.[13]

Most studies linking hormone replacement therapy with breast cancer use premarin and provera, which are not bio-identical hormones. Our detoxification system plays an important role in cancer prevention. Premarin® blocks the important Phase II detoxification enzyme, glutathione S-transferase.[16] This blocking action of a critical detoxification step helps explain why Premarin® does not show the same breast protective effect that estradiol does. Studies have also shown that metabolites of equine estrogens cause oxidative damage to DNA, which also helps explain how long term use of Premarin® is linked to breast cancer.[17]

Progesterone

Progesterone appears to be an anti-breast cancer hormone. Several studies have been published that support the existence of this effect.

- A prospective epidemiological study done at Johns Hopkins Hospital demonstrated the protective role of natural progesterone against breast cancer. They followed 1,083 women who were evaluated and treated for infertility for thirteen to thirty-three years. The results showed that the breast cancer rate was almost five and a half times higher in women who had a lower progesterone level compared to those with a normal progesterone level.[18]

- Application of progesterone gel to the breast has been shown to reduce the growth activity of the breast glands.[19]

- Studies have demonstrated that in progesterone receptor positive breast cancer cells, progesterone regulates the gene expression and results in cancer cell death. [20,21,22]

It must be emphasized only bio-identical progesterone had those anti-cancer effects, not synthetic progestins like medroxyprogesterone. Unfortunately, most medical literature does not distinguish between natural and synthetic progesterone and most physicians believe progesterone and progestins are the same thing, when in fact, the minimal change in the natural molecules that transform it into a progestin changes the entire action and function of the molecule.

We also know estrogen helps with good health in the areas of mood, memory, blood pressure, and the cardiovascular system. So why did the WHI study produce such discouraging results as increased cardiovascular complications, stroke, and dementia? It is very likely that some of the complications were related to the use of edroxyprogesterone (a synthetic progestin), rather than bio-identical progesterone.

- Articles show that medroxyprogesterone increases the progression of coronary artery heart disease and causes insulin resistance and subsequent hyperglycemia.[23, 24] Both of these outcomes are related to diabetes.

- In a study published in *The American Journal of Cardiology*, researchers studied two groups of postmenopausal women who had coronary heart disease. Both groups used estradiol (E2) for two weeks, then one group received intravaginal progesterone and the other group received oral progestin. Treadmill exercise tests were performed before hormone treatment as a baseline, two weeks after use of estradiol alone, and then at ten days after adding progesterone or progestin. The study found that patients exercised on the treadmill longer without chest pain (myocardial ischemia) when they took two weeks of estradiol compared to their baselines. After adding bio-identical progesterone, the benefit of longer exercise time persisted, but with the use of synthetic progestin the benefit disappeared.[25]

Testosterone

Testosterone has been shown to have a direct anti-breast cancer effect. Consider the evidence below:

- A NIH (National Institutes of Health) study demonstrated that testosterone decreases the activities of breast cancer cells in monkeys.[26]
- In Italy, researchers demonstrated that testosterone inhibits breast cancer cells through it is own hormone receptor.[27]

In a clinical setting, this means the addition of testosterone, along with progesterone, has the benefit of breast cancer protection. However, if someone has a very high aromatase enzyme in the breast which converts testosterone into estrogen, the situation may be different.

DHEA

Low DHEA levels have been associated with higher breast cancer risk in pre- menopausal women; on the other hand, high DHEA levels have also been associated with a higher incidence of breast cancer.[28] So for the time being, the best strategy is to keep DHEA levels within the normal range.

Melatonin

Melatonin is not just a sleep hormone; it also has anti-inflammation and anti-cancer effects. Night shift workers, such as nurses, tend to have lower melatonin levels and higher rates of breast cancer.[29] Using melatonin in a physiological dose should be considered in all women suffering from insomnia.

Many women are afraid to use HRT and will choose to suffer and have a low or poor quality of life and continuous battles with age related diseases. The actual causes of breast cancer are compromised immune systems due to stress and excessive toxins that can trigger inflammation. Balanced hormone therapy does not increase the rate of breast cancer and may even help to reduce it. Bio-identical hormone therapy can help you sleep better which improves your immune system and thus reduce the risk of cancer. It can improve your moods and memory and thus improve your quality of life.

Hormone Replacement Therapy – Routes of Delivery

Not all hormone replacement therapies are created equal. Although they all claim to treat menopausal symptoms, the way that they go about doing it can differ widely, not just in formulation (natural vs. synthetic), but also in the way they are applied and maintained. For the informed individual seeking relief from menopausal and mid-life hormonal deficiencies, the secret to success is finding a safe and effective method of hormone replacement.

Routes of Delivery Options

1. Oral—

    a. When taking any medication orally, it is first absorbed in the GI (gastrointestinal) tract, after which 90 percent of the medicine goes directly to and excreted by the liver. This is known as "first-pass metabolism."

    b. Before menopause, our ovaries secrete hormones directly into the bloodstream through the capillaries. These hormones do not go to the liver first. Rather, they go directly to wherever they are needed in the body, undiluted and at full-strength. It is only after the body has used what it needs that any excess hormones are sent to the liver for excretion.

    c. Estrogen taken orally reverses this normal route of hormone metabolism. The liver sequesters so much in its attempt of detoxifying the hormones; higher doses are required than our body actually needs in order to have a high enough concentration in the blood for the medication to do the job.

d.   Additionally, estrogen taken orally increases the inflammation and clotting factors made in the liver. Studies have shown that bypassing the oral route with transdermal or implanted hormones does not negatively impact these cardiovascular risk factors.[30,31] These consequences reveal why taking estrogen orally is not the best way to receive hormone replacement.

2.   Transdermal—

a.   Transdermal methods of delivery involve direct application to the skin. This is usually accomplished by using hormone creams, gels, or patches. Currently two bioequivalent estrogen (E2) patches (Vivelle-Dot® and Climara®) have been made available. A transdermal form of the bio-equivalent progesterone patch has not yet been developed. Testosterone patches are available for men, but not for women. One drawback of patches is that they have adhesives which can cause skin irritation. Creams or gels have to be applied at least once a day, and they can be messy. Compliance is a concern, since people tend to forget to apply the cream, particularly if their memories are not very good. Absorption is another issue, which is affected by each individual's skin condition and the mixing substance used to manufacture the cream or gel. Creams can be useful for women if their skin absorption is adequate and they remember to consistently apply the cream.

3.   Sublingual—

a.   Sublingual lozenges or troches under the tongue deliver hormones directly through the mucosa in the mouth. The sublingual route of delivery causes a surge of hormones which diminishes within eight to twelve hours. Many people cannot handle this surge of hormones.

b.   Progesterone is the only hormone I give my patients in the sublingual form, since our body had progesterone only 50 percent of the time in our younger years. With the calming effect, it helps people sleep at night and the level goes down in the daytime thus does not cause drowsiness during the day.

4.   Suppositories—

a.   Intravaginal or rectal suppositories can also be used to deliver hormones, but due to the discomfort involved many women dislike this route.

5.   Injections—

a.   Intramuscular injections cause a surge of hormones which diminishes quickly and require weekly or monthly injections. A significant drawback with this method of delivery is that bio-identical hormones are not available for injections.

6.   Subcutaneous (beneath the skin) Pellet Implants—

a.   This is the most physiologically appropriate form of hormone replacement. It is as if your own ovaries are functioning again. The many benefits of this route of hormone replacement are discussed in detail in Chapter 4.

The following chart, figure 4, illustrates the absorbability of different hormone delivery routes. As you can see, pellet implants have the greatest absorption over the long-term.

Hormone Routes and Absorbability

Fol = Follicular
Ov = Ovulatory
Lut = Luteal
Memo = Menopausal

Mean hormone concentrations achieved with different routes of estrogen delivery. (Englund, et al., 1977; Thom, et al., 1981; Powers, et al., 1985; Garnett, et al., 1990; Stanczyck, 1991).

Source: Studd JW and Smith RN. Oestradiol and testosterone implants. *Baillières Clin Endocrinol Metab.* 1993;7(1):203-223. Reprinted with permission.

Figure 4.   Mean hormone concentrations.

Rules of Hormone Replacement

The use of hormone replacement therapy requires paying attention to important details. Here are the guidelines:

    1.   If you need hormone replacement, use bio-identical hormones that are delivered through physiological routes, such as through the skin or implanted beneath the skin.

2.   Remember that all of the body's hormones are interrelated. It is important to balance all hormones, including the sex, adrenal, and thyroid hormones.

3.   Hormone levels must be monitored periodically to make sure they are balanced and in the appropriate normal ranges. There have been many studies published on hormone replacement therapy, The Women's Health Initiative Study being one of the most influential. Even though it produced negative results for the reasons we discussed earlier, many studies conducted in the past have demonstrated the ability of HRT to reduce heart disease and dementia. There are currently many ongoing studies of HRT, and when the cloud of dust from all the research finally settles in the next twenty to thirty years, I believe that the positive results we are seeing today will continue to be validated.

Women who use the right type of hormone replacement will experience an improved quality of life into their golden years by reducing heart disease, strokes, dementia, and osteoporosis. This is in addition to the benefits of reducing hot flashes, improving sleep, mood, memory, libido, and energy – after all, isn't this what every man and woman wants?

Chapter 4

Subcutaneous Bio-identical Hormone Pellet Implants

The Ultimate Hormone Replacement Therapy

The first documented instance of an implant for hormone replacement occurred in 1938 at Guy's Hospital in London. It was developed at that time for women who had undergone a radical hysterectomy (removal of uterus) and bilateral oophorectomy (removal of both ovaries). In spite of many apparent advantages over other delivery routes, such as oral medications or gels or patches, hormone pellets are only used by a few trained physicians in English-speaking countries such as the United Kingdom, Australia, South Africa, and the United States. Physicians are trained to use hormone replacement therapy in the United States relying on hormone pills and patches manufactured and promoted by pharmaceutical companies. Many doctors are biased against bio-identical hormones and most doctors have not even heard about pellet therapy, but assume they are just as bad as synthetic hormones, which does not appear to be true.

Advantages of Pellet Therapy Demonstrated in Studies

In England Dr. John Studd published many papers on pellet implants and argued the hormone profiles achieved and the efficacy of implant therapy should be used as a first-line therapy in patients with severe menopausal symptoms.[32,33]

His studies, as well as others showed:

1. There was no evidence linking pellet therapy to an increased incidence of breast cancer.[34]

.2. Orally administered estrogen is associated with altered coagulation factors and lipid panels while subcutaneously implanted pellets show no adverse effect on blood pressure, lipids, coagulation factors, and insulin and glucose metabolism.[35,36,37] As discussed in the previous chapter, this is because the subcutaneous implantation of hormone pellets bypasses the liver and avoids the induction of liver factors that can negatively impact the cardiovascular system.

3. Pellet therapy restores the 2:1 ratio E2 to E1, which is the physiological balance of younger age women, and effectively improves bone density when compared to other methods of hormone replacement. Studd et al. There was a demonstrated four-fold increase (8.3%) in bone density in patients who received pellets compared to oral estrogen (2.8%) in postmenopausal women after one year of treatment.[38]

4. Pellet therapy promotes a more stable blood level compared to pills and patches. Oral estrogen has a roller coaster effect, while the patch is more stable but still goes up and down. Pellets are the only delivery method that provides stable E2 blood levels.

    a. Montgomery et al. demonstrated that estradiol implants were significantly more effective than placebo in relieving depression and anxiety in postmenopausal women.[39]

    b. Testosterone implants help to improve libido and weight loss by building muscles. Other types of HRT usually do not use testosterone. Transdermal testosterone cream does not achieve the same results as implanted pellets.

    c. Pellet therapy is hassle free; there are no creams to rub on every day or patches to replace once or twice a week.

Blood Level Comparisons of Pellet Implants, Patch, and Oral

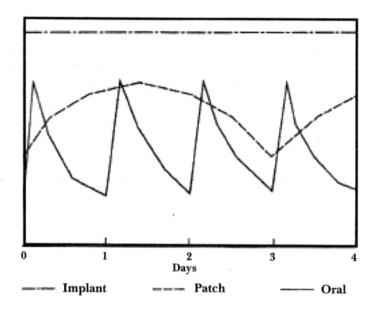

Figure 5. Short-term variation in estradiol concentrations with pellet implant, patch, and oral therapy.

Source: Studd JW and Smith RN. Oestradiol and testosterone implants. *Baillières Clin Endocrinol Metab.* 1993;7(1):203-223. Reprinted with permission.

Source: Studd JW and Smith RN. Oestradiol and testosterone implants. Baillieres Clin Endocrinol Metab. 1993;7(1):203-223. Reprinted with permission.

Implant Procedure

Implanting pellets is an easy, quick, and safe office procedure carried out under local anesthesia, so there is minimal to no pain involved. The skin is cleansed with an antiseptic and then numbed. A tiny incision (3 mm) is made and the pellets are inserted through a trochar (tool used to inject pellet) just under the skin, into the subcutaneous fat of either the lower abdominal wall or the outer quarter of the buttock. Afterward the incision is covered with a sterile strip. A stitch may be required only if there is excessive bleeding.

Biological Action of Implants

After implantation, there is a rapid rise of estradiol and a decline of follicular stimulating hormone (FSH), which is a hormone secreted by the pituitary gland to regulate estrogen. A high level of FSH means the body wants to stimulate the ovaries to produce more estrogen. A lower FSH level means the body feels that there is enough estrogen, so the ovaries do not need to be stimulated to make more.

The figures below show the decline in FSH and rise in E1 and E2 after a 50 mg pellet implantation, which is then followed by their respective gradual rise and fall.

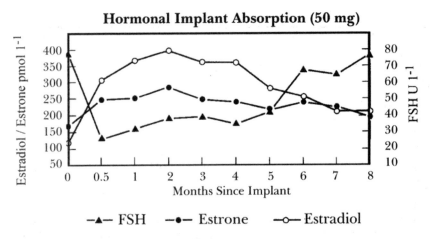

Figure 6.   FSH, estrone and estradiol concentrations with 50 mg estradiol implant.

Source: Studd JW and Smith RN. Oestradiol and testosterone implants. Baillieres Clin Endocrinol Metab. 1993;7(1):203-223. Reprinted with permission.

Frequently Asked Questions

1.   How soon will I see the effects of pellet therapy? How long do the pellets last and how will I know when the pellets begin to run out?

a. My patients usually see effects within one week, some even in one to two days. The amount of time pellets last can vary with the individual, but it is usually between four to six months. While the original symptoms might not return together all at once, they will gradually reappear one-by-one, alerting patients to the fact that it is time for an implant again.

2. How does the body know to take the proper amount of hormones it needs?

a. Since a hormone pellet is surrounded by blood vessels under the skin, its rate of hormone release is regulated by the heart rate and cardiac output (the amount of blood pumped out of the heart with a single contraction), also the size of the pellet. Imagine a sand stone in the river, each time the water runs through the stone, it rubs on the surface of the stone and carries away a little sand. The slower the water runs through the stone, the less sand is being released. The bigger the stone, the more sand will be released. The slower the heart rate the fewer hormones are released. Therefore, more hormones are released when the heart rate rises with either physical or emotional stress. When the physical (exercise, strenuous work) or emotional stress is no longer present the amount of hormone released from the pellet will decrease and return to the steady continuous flow provided by a normal heart rate.

b. The amount of hormone released is also dependent upon both the dosage as well as the hormone concentration difference between the pellet and blood vessel. A higher dosage (a larger sized pellet) provides a greater contact surface that releases more hormones to the blood stream. A hormonally depleted body will also pull more hormones from the pellet since the concentration in the blood stream will be lower than the tissue surrounding the pellet.

c. With this method of hormonal delivery, the tissue hormone levels are stable twenty-four hours a day, seven days a week. Because the estrogen levels do not go too high or fluctuate, pellet therapy does not stimulate the breasts at the same level as synthetic hormones.

d.   If a person is stressed and the body requires the support of more hormones, the pellets will be used more quickly. It is similar to having a full tank of gas in the car. If you drive a lot, the tank will empty sooner. This is the only form of hormone therapy that can deliver more as needed.

3.   What is in the pellets?

a.   Pellets are made of bio-identical estradiol or testosterone. They are made in different dosages by compounding pharmacies; fused into the size of a grain of rice, sterilized, and stored in individual small glass containers. Progesterone should not be implanted because a woman's natural menstrual cycle only provides progesterone 50 percent of the time, not the 100 percent of the time an implanted pellet would supply.

4.   Is it FDA approved?

a.   A testosterone pellet called Testopel has recently been approved by the FDA. Bio-identical estradiol is approved by the FDA and currently made by compounding pharmacists who operate at all times with federal and state mandated guidelines.

5.   Will my period return when I am on pellet therapy?

a.   If your estrogen returns to levels you had at a younger age, and you use progesterone for only two weeks out of the month, you will have a period. It can actually be a good idea to have a period, as it helps to clean up the uterine linings. However, if you do not want to have your period back, take progesterone continuously as this suppresses the growth of the uterus lining and will prevent the occurrence of a period.

Indications for Pellet Therapy

Let us take a look now at some of the primary conditions and their symptoms that indicate a person's need for hormone replacement. Individual patient stories will also help to illustrate the effectiveness of pellet therapy in treating these conditions.

1.   Menopause—
   a.   The most common reason that women seek hormone replacement therapy is due to menopausal symptoms. These include:
      i.   Hot flashes and/or night sweats
      ii.   Insomnia or poor quality of sleep
      iii.   Fatigue
      iv.   Moodiness
      v.   Depression and/or anxiety
      vi.   Memory loss/forgetfulness
      vii.   Difficulty concentrating
      viii.   Lack of motivation
      ix.   Heart palpitations
      x.   Hair loss
      xi.   Vaginal dryness, painful intercourse, low libido
      xii.   Urinary incontinence or infection
      xiii.   Aching joints and muscles
      xiv.   Bone loss/osteoporosis
   b.   All of these symptoms due to low hormone levels are relieved when implanted pellets deliver adequate hormone replacement.

2.   Perimenopause—Laurie's story:

My name is Laurie, age fifty, and a few years ago I became perimenopausal, which started with hot flashes that would wake me up at 3:30 or so every morning. I also noticed that I had no tolerance or patience for things that had not previously bothered me. Headaches and joint pains also started to occur. Since my older sister had already been going through menopause, I was aware that my symptoms meant I was in its early stages.

I am proactive about my health, including being very diligent about nutrition and exercising regularly. I was aware that weight gain usually comes with menopause. While that had not happened to me yet, I was concerned about it. So, I began reading books about menopause and found out about a hormone saliva test to determine if I was menopausal. My efforts to find someone to administer this test led me to Karen Sun, M.D. Sure enough, the test showed that I was indeed perimenopausal.

Other symptoms that had set in included less confidence and a lack of mental clarity. Until I became perimenopausal, I had been a very confident person, but suddenly I doubted myself on things that before I knew were a given. Things just no longer were making sense in my life. It is like in those commercials where the bird flies into the window. That is kind of how it feels being perimenopausal. Dr. Sun and I decided to go with the pellets to alleviate my symptoms. After I had the pellets, I suddenly felt better. My frame of mind improved. I had more strength when I worked out at the gym, and the hormones balanced things out.

They have helped me get through the hills and valleys of life a lot more easily. It was as though one day someone lifted the shade that had covered my life. When you get your hormones right, everything becomes crystal clear, and I wondered why I had struggled with all that stuff before.

A female colleague talked about being perimenopausal, how there is nothing you can do about it, and that there is nothing you can take to feel better. I told her that is not true and talked with her about what Dr. Sun had done for me. We do not have to be miserable; we do not have to go through hot flashes, insomnia, or weight gain if we have pellets. I try to tell as many people about this as possible.

I recently had my skin evaluated for a special facial treatment, and the lady told me that I do not look anywhere near fifty. She said, "Whatever you are doing, keep doing it." I think the hormones preserve us all the way around. I feel lucky that my research took me in the direction of Dr. Sun.

I want to be happy; I don't want to be miserable. I feel very blessed that I have been able to find Dr. Sun and experience this relief from menopausal symptoms. She has made my life so much better. She has put her heart and soul into helping her patients get their hormones balanced. I know she has changed the lives of many. I know for a fact that she has improved my quality of life.

When a woman is perimenopausal, or at the early stage of entering menopause, she will still have a menstrual period, but it will be very irregular. Hot flashes may or may not occur. The most bothersome symptoms are moodiness, especially immediately prior to the menstrual period; migraine headaches; and sleep disturbance. These symptoms are due to the fluctuation of hormone levels, especially when a woman is stressed and her body is not able to produce higher levels of hormones to meet the increased need.

I find that pellet implants with testosterone alone are very helpful in this situation, because testosterone stabilizes the estrogen levels by converting to estrogen at the cellular level. Testosterone is also very effective in relieving moodiness, low libido, and fatigue symptoms, which happen quite often at this stage. In many women the same symptoms are treated with birth control pills, but the results achieved through implanted pellets are much more effective. If there is heavy bleeding or breast tenderness present, I will add progesterone cream or lozenges to address these symptoms.

3.   Menstrual Migraines—Erica's story:

My name is Erica, and I started getting very severe migraines during my second pregnancy, which happened seven years ago. The headaches worsened progressively thereafter and typically occurred around my menstrual cycle. My doctor and the specialists to whom I had been referred put me on a lot of different medications, including injections and antidepressants.

Nonetheless, I was still having migraine headaches that were so terrible they made me vomit. I even had to go to the hospital a couple of times. These headaches put me out of commission. They would last for days, and I was completely not functioning in life. I thought I was going to have to quit work, and I could not even take care of my children. Then I read a book called The Hormone Solution, which is when I first heard about bio-identical hormones. At the time I lived in Connecticut and flew to California to see Dr. Sun. I was in very bad shape, but within a few days of having the pellets my migraines abated, and I have not had a terrible migraine since. I have been able to go off of all the medications, including the antidepressants. The pellets have been the total miracle cure for me. I have been on the pellets for two years now, and I have my life back. To be able to play with my kids again and function in life is really awesome.

Migraines are a common disorder affecting about 20 percent of all women. The fact that migraines usually start after puberty and 60 percent of these headaches are related to the menstrual period suggests that this is a hormone issue. I also find that testosterone implants are helpful for this condition, as it stabilizes the hormone levels. I have quite a few patients suffering from menstrual migraines who have tried other treatments without effect. Testosterone pellet implantation often helps them tremendously, as well as very small doses of estradiol in pellet form.

4.   Osteoporosis—Amelia's story:

I am Amelia, sixty-three, with a slender build and of Scandinavian descent. All of these factors are typical risks for osteoporosis. I went for my first bone density exam about twelve years ago. I was told at that time that I have thinning bones. So, I was put on various medications for this condition. Each year as I would have a bone density scan and would find out that my condition sometimes was better, or worse, depending on the type of medication I had been given. Then came the scare about taking estrogen, so I went off of it and used a hormone replacement therapy in the form of a cream. I also wanted to go off of the bone density medication after a CT scan showed that I had a lot of liver cysts.

This was when I went to Dr. Sun, who introduced me to the possibility of pellets. She is in favor of using the physiological route of delivery of bio-identical hormones by subcutaneous implantation instead of the oral delivery through the stomach and liver. I decided to try the pellets for a year to see what would happen. I received estrogen and testosterone pellets and sublingual progesterone. After a year, my bone density exam showed an increase of bone density in my hip and spine. This increase had to be as a result of the pellets, as this was the only thing I was doing differently. Other bone meds will keep down deterioration of bone but do not build new bone. Now I have had between 1.4% and 2.1% increases in bone density in various areas. What is more, my liver function has tested as normal. This is very encouraging.

Both estrogen and testosterone improve bone density. Pellet implant therapy supplies the body with a steady amount of hormones so it is more effective than other routes of hormone therapy in treating osteoporosis.

5.   Depression and Anxiety—Vicki's story:

I am Vicki, sixty-seven, and I have been very healthy and active all my life, working out and playing tennis until age fifty. I was running six miles a day. Then, menopause struck. My worst symptom was anxiety. I was married at the time to a physician who did not believe in hormone replacement therapy. He said it was unnatural and that I should just tough it out. Being the good wife, that is what I did. I have not been the type to be anxious and stay at home, but I became that way. I was afraid and very unsure of myself. Then, my husband died when I was fifty-three. I became so anxious that it came to the point I could not function. It was a terrible time in my life. I sold my husband's medical practice to another physician, who told me to get on hormones. He started giving me synthetic estrogen injections. That worked all right for a few years until the controversy over hormones occurred. Even that doctor said then that I should get off the hormones. I finally stopped them and then I really started to feel bad. I had no libido; I became super anxious; I had no energy at all. I just dragged through the day. This went on for a full year until I found out about bio-identical hormone replacement therapy.

After I went on the pellets, I started to feel so much better and I became a different person. I had no more anxiety, and I was stronger. I went back to being the way I was before menopause. The pellets have been tremendous. I am so rejuvenated and I have absolutely no side effects. I am back to playing golf, swimming, and walking at least four miles a day. All of my anxiety and other symptoms were a result of the lack of hormones. Once we got that under control, I became fine. This is wonderful. I feel healthy and good. I will continue to do this until I die.

The role of hormones in depression is well documented in patients with postpartum (after childbirth) depression and premenstrual syndrome. Pellet implants improve mood, especially depression and anxiety. In my clinical experience I have seen many patients who have been treated with antidepressants or tranquilizers before they have come to me. After pellet implantation, I have often been able to help them reduce or discontinue antidepressants and tranquilizers successfully.

6. Testosterone Deficiency and Sexual Dysfunction— Carey's Story:

My name is Carey, forty-seven, and for a couple of years before I found the pellets, I was absolutely uninterested in sex. Period. End of story. Any lovemaking I did with my husband was from a sense of duty. Now, with my hormones at a normal, healthy level, I have more of a sex drive. I no longer have to accept that losing interest in my sexuality is unavoidable and a part of growing older. I like feeling attractive and sensual again. It is great to have regained this special connection with my husband. I also like the mental clarity and getting up in the morning feeling rested. I like waking up with energy. Those are the benefits I feel from the pellets more than anything else.

Most women are embarrassed to admit how low libido bothers them. After pellet therapy, many women have told me that they have experienced such dramatic improvements in their sex lives that their husbands have talked about sending me flowers. Their husbands, in fact, are usually the ones who remind them they are due for pellets. Women, who once had no interest in dating, experience such a boost in their libido and self-confidence that they completely reinvigorated their social lives; in many cases they start dating and even get married after receiving pellet treatment.

Female Androgen Insufficiency Syndrome (FAIS) widely exists but is rarely talked about. So far, it is a clinical diagnosis made from signs and symptoms. The clinical symptoms of FAIS include decreased libido and sexual pleasure, a diminished sense of well-being, depressed mood or lack of motivation, and persistent fatigue. Physical signs include bone loss, decreased muscle mass and reduced strength, which leads to more fat in the body.

The normal level for testosterone in women has not been well established. Pre-menopausal women produce 0.1 to 0.2 mg of testosterone daily and to maintain the normal function of the human body, women must receive the equivalent amount of testosterone when receiving hormone therapy. Most labs use a normal value of 20 to 80 ng/dl, which is outdated. In a paper published out of Princeton University Medical School, a number of the world's experts on testosterone therapy for women found that all the assays used most frequently by the laboratories could not measure levels of testosterone below 300 ng/dl accurately.[40]

Additionally, hormone levels vary in different age groups, and no normal values for different age groups have been established. Furthermore, most testosterone is bound up with hormone-binding protein, and only the unbound component (free testosterone) is active. Testosterone testing is designed for men who have ten times more testosterone than women. So, this test becomes inaccurate when the free testosterone is measured at women's much lower levels. Another factor not often accounted for is the possibility of testosterone resistance, like insulin resistance, which can affect the interpretation of test results. One may show sufficient hormone levels in a blood test but still have the symptoms of deficiency.

I find the most common cause of FAIS is adrenal fatigue. Remember, the adrenal glands secrete DHEA, which is the precursor to testosterone. Most women are so stressed in their daily lives that almost all of them suffer from adrenal fatigue, just with varying degrees of severity. Another reason for FAIS is surgical oophorectomy (removal of an ovary or both ovaries) or incidental injury to blood circulation in the ovaries due to other surgeries, such as hysterectomy or tubal ligation. By suppressing ovulation and reducing FSH (follicular stimulation hormone), birth control pills result in reduced production of testosterone from the ovaries.

7.   Adrenal Fatigue—Sarah's story:

I am Sarah, seventy-four, a retired college professor. I was experiencing increasing exhaustion, and when I read up on the adrenals I thought they could be a factor in my being so tired. Then I had three serious operations on my knees and neck over a two and a half year period. I became so tired, had no energy, was depressed, and cried constantly. Everything was a monumental effort, and I am a high-energy person. When I walked into Dr. Sun's office a year ago, I was wiped out. My head was literally crouched over the steering wheel of my car. She could see that I was hanging by a thread. She gave me a small pellet insertion and we went from there. Little by little, she has brought me back to health. The pellets are a miracle, and I could not live without them. I have been on them for a year now and never want to be without them again. We are working on building up my adrenals with the combination of pellets and supplemental medications, such as hydrocortisone and adrenal herbs. I do feel more energy and have more zest for life. This has been an incredible transformation, as I am now taking water aerobics classes and working in my garden again.

The reduced functioning of the adrenal glands is a modern disease due primarily to chronic stress and longer lifetimes. In Chapter 7 we will be talking about this epidemic in detail. I find that pellet therapy with testosterone is very helpful in relieving the symptoms of fatigue. Testosterone is one of the major sources of estrogen for women after menopause, since testosterone can convert into estrogen in the tissue. When women have their ovaries removed, they have a more difficult time coping with menopausal symptoms because after menopause the body depends on the ovarian production of testosterone. The same holds true for women who have adrenal fatigue, because decreased production of DHEA by the adrenal glands also results in low levels of testosterone.

8.   Cystitis and Urinary Tract Infection—Andrea's story:

I am Andrea, aged fifty-nine, and I have had interstitial cystitis (IC), or painful bladder syndrome, for twenty-five years. This disease causes the pain and symptoms of a urinary tract infection, but it is not caused by bacteria. A million people in the U.S. have this disease, and 80 to 90 percent are female. Urologists have been searching for the answers for what causes IC. It is something wrong with the lining of the bladder. It certainly is life altering. Many people cannot work or leave their homes because of this disease. In many cases, it leads to suicide. It is just dreadful. I am lucky that my symptoms are moderate to severe, and I have a high tolerance for pain, but this disease has been the bane of my existence.

It comes on periodically. It hurts to urinate with IC; it is like being allergic to your own urine, and you have to go to the bathroom constantly. When I was diagnosed twenty-five years ago, the only treatment was a bladder wash that instills DMSO (dimethyl sulfoxide). It can bring relief, and I have had DMSO once every six weeks to two months. Then a new drug called Elmiron came out. Although it helps with IC symptoms, it can make you lose your hair. I like my hair, so I did not continue with this drug. For fifteen years I have been on Elavil, an antidepressant that has the amazing benefit of blocking pain. I have kept the symptoms of IC reasonably under control with these three treatments. I also had a hysterectomy around the same time I was diagnosed with IC, and one ovary was removed two years later. At first I was on Estrace® for hormone replacement therapy and then switched to another form of estradiol after a couple of years.

None of these hormone therapies made any difference at all with the IC symptoms. It never occurred to me to connect hormones with this disease. But when I started on the implanted bio-identical hormone pellet therapy with Dr. Sun a few years ago, all of my IC symptoms were suddenly reduced by about 70 percent. It was absolutely unbelievable. After the pellets were implanted, I went six months without DMSO bladder irrigation. Then I went ten months without it. Naturally, I said something to my urologist about this link. He said he was not surprised because hormone therapy helps support the bladder. I cannot tell you the difference the pellet therapy has made in my life. I love the pellets for all the other obvious reasons. Everything is better with the pellets, but I would use them if for no other reason than they have changed the nature of this disease that I have had. My urologist gives women hormone creams, but that does not do it like the pellets. I tried them. There is something very different about the pellets that make them so much more effective. In addition, they make me feel more youthful.

Having provided pellet therapy to over 1,000 patients now, coupled with Dr. Tutera treating over 10,000 patients, we have both witnessed an amazing number of success stories. Andrea, with interstitial cystitis, is just one example. Some of my patients have tried multiple antidepressants without relief, only to find that pellet therapy is the only thing that alleviates their depression. Women suffering from fibromyalgia improve greatly with pellet therapy. Other women burdened by adrenal fatigue recovered after their sleeping patterns improved due to pellet therapy. The list of benefits goes on and on.

Best Candidates for Pellet Therapy

The following categories describe those groups of women who are generally best suited to benefit from pellet therapy.

1. Women who have adrenal fatigue and become surgically menopausal with removal of both ovaries and the uterus.

Elizabeth's story—

My journey began when I entered perimenopause at the age of forty. I now know that I was entering it early as my job was very demanding, and I was in a stage of adrenal fatigue, as well as only had one functioning ovary. My primary symptom was very heaving bleeding with many clots being passed.
    Even though I had been in the medical profession my whole life, I did not understand my body well enough to know that it was progesterone that was lacking and natural progesterone would have probably corrected the problem. Instead, I believed my doctor that estrogen would help and took the oral cotradiol he prescribed. Over a course of three years the bleeding never improved, and he told me that a hysterectomy was my only answer. I sought out a female gynecologist for a second opinion, and did not realize that doctors are trained with the same medical school training, as she agreed a hysterectomy was the

only answer and told me, I would "feel better than ever afterwards." I trusted both of these opinions, especially since they agreed with each other, and at the age of forty-three agreed to a hysterectomy. When I woke up with an estrogen pill being shoved down my throat, I found out the doctor also took my ovaries even though he had never once discussed this with me. When I asked why he took them, he told me, "Well you are over forty and you don't want cancer in your future, do you?" I realized I could not put my ovaries back, so I went home determined to feel so much better than ever afterwards.

Over the weeks and month that followed, however, I did not. I fell into a deep, suicidal depression, my blood pressure was out of control even though it had been low normal my entire life, I had no energy and even quit going to work as all I could do was drag my body around all day, and sexually had lost all feeling and ability to respond. When I told my doctor about all these symptoms, he told me it was all in my head and wanted to refer me to a psychiatrist. When I said, no this was a chemical change, he referred me to an endocrinologist who just changed my brand of oral estrogen and added progesterone cream.

After a year and half, I finally found a doctor who understood the symptoms caused by the loss of my ovaries. She explained that I was not absorbing the oral estrogen and she felt about 20 percent of women do not. She also helped me understand I must have been a high testosterone maker and was missing the testosterone as much, if not more than, the estrogen. As a result, she started me on a combination of estradiol and testosterone shots. These would make me feel like my old self for only about a day, so I was getting shots once a week. We tried estradiol and testosterone creams. These did not help me feel any better. She also explained that some women do not absorb creams, so I was one of those also. Then we tried the estradiol patches. I never felt good on them and was swimming every day and I found they just floated off into the pool. After a year and a half of working with her and still not feeling good, she said there was a company that was attempting to get FDA approval for hormone pellet implants. She explained they were compact pure hormone pellets that would be implanted under the skin. I was ready to try anything at this time, as I had not felt good the entire three years since my surgery. Even though I did not feel their effect for two weeks, when I finally started feeling their effect, I was elated, as it was the first time since surgery that I felt anywhere near close to my old self. That was in 1988 and I have been on them almost consistently since then. There was a two year period of time when the company that made the pellets went bankrupt, and I could not obtain them anymore. I tried several other manufacturers of the pellets but was not absorbing them. At the time, I went back to the shots, the creams, and the patches, and fell into all the same horrific symptoms I had felt after surgery. I was hot flashing and crying on a daily basis. Again I had no energy and no ability to respond sexually. At this time I also developed the excruciatingly painful symptoms of fibromyalgia as well as had osteoarthritis in my hands, which was so bad I could not hold hands with my husband and my joints had taken on the gnarled misshapen appearance of arthritic joints. I finally called my family practitioner and said, "You have got to find pellets for me. They are the only things that work for me." She found the pellets and within two weeks after implanting them the hot flashes, crying, and my fibromyalgia disappeared totally. I was thrilled to feel good again and to understand that the fibromyalgia had been connected to just low estradiol and testosterone. Four months later I also realized the pain in the joints in my hands had disappeared. I was delighted with this and did not expect my joints to return to their normal shape. However, two years after being on consistent pellet implantations I realized all the joints in my fingers had returned to normal shape and size. I was equally thrilled to realize this condition was not an inevitable outcome of growing old; it was only that my body needed estradiol and testosterone in order for the joints to stay healthy.

After using the pellets for eighteen years, Dr. Sun convinced me to increase my testosterone dosage, even though it was out of range for normal women. I am so thankful she understood this, as the increased dosage finally restored my sexual response to what it was before surgery. Up until that time, the pellet dose had brought the response back to 80 percent. I did not think to question it, as I was thrilled to feel anything, as I did not without the pellet implants. Now, twenty years of almost consistent pellet implants makes me a believer in them, and has given me the understanding that women do not have to suffer with what we have thought were inevitable conditions of growing old. These conditions arise out of our loss of estradiol at menopause and for those of us who have had the misfortune of having our ovaries removed, the loss of testosterone also. I know when my pellets are running out. I marvel at how the body knows better than we do what it needs to maintain proper functioning. When my pellets start running low, I start in with problems with my memory and my ability to put thoughts together cohesively. I also start getting vertigo and become incontinent. Hot flashes can start and I start becoming more emotional and depressed, as well as start sleeping less and sometimes have night sweats. In addition, I have found that when my body is stressed, because it utilizes them at a much greater rate, I need to have the implants more often.

The difference in my quality of life is so profound that I know that I do not ever want to function again without having these precious, vitally important hormones replaced about every four months. I celebrate the doctors who utilized them in the beginning and all the doctors who have been open to realizing that pellets are a Godsend for women who do not absorb hormones readily and need them in order to function on a daily basis.

Elizabeth's story is not unusual. Many women have the same story. This is the worst situation that can occur when women who are already suffering from adrenal fatigue suddenly become surgically menopausal. These women develop severe menopausal symptoms, even to the point of suicidal depression and have difficulty carrying out daily activities. Many women have gone from doctor to doctor seeking help, only to be put on antidepressants, sleeping pills, and all kinds of less effective hormone therapies that bring no relief. As previously observed and supported by research, subcutaneously implanted bio-identical hormone therapy is optimally effective and should be offered as a first-line therapy to avoid suffering and deterioration of health. Unfortunately, a good majority of gynecologists are unfamiliar with pellet therapy and, therefore, patients are not offered this option.

2. Women who have had a hysterectomy and/or oophorectomy, especially women younger than forty-five years old.

Erica's story—

My name is Erica; I am fifty-two years old. When I was sixteen, I became pregnant for the first time, and I had drastic mood swings. By the time I was in my twenties, I was one of those women who could kill somebody at that time of the month. For about two weeks each month, I was like that. I don't know how my husband stayed with me, because I was horrible. At age thirty-one, after having three children, I had to have a hysterectomy. When I awoke the next morning, I thought the room was excessively hot. The nurse told me that I was probably having hot flashes. I was immediately thrown into menopause, even though I still had my ovaries. I talked with the doctor about the hot flashes, and he suggested that I use hormones. After a few different treatments without help, he told me about bio-identical hormone pellets. I was desperate, and he put in the hormone implant. Within four to five days, I noticed a big difference in my life. My mood was even and my sex drive was back, which I had lost after the hysterectomy. My concentration was better. My doctor told me that the pellets help your bones and skin. I continued to get those implants. I'm now fifty-two and I've been getting the pellets for well over twenty years. I have ten times more energy than other women my age. And I have an excitement about life. The pellets help me to keep evenly keeled and to think straight. I no longer have huge emotional dips. If a woman starts talking about symptoms of menopause, and her husband says that his wife has turned into a witch overnight, I tell them about the implants. People have told me I have saved their marriages. The implants are my life, literally. If I don't have them, I know I won't have any quality of life.

3.   Menopausal women who are symptomatic and have not responded to other treatments.

4.   Women who are perimenopausal and experience hormone fluctuations and are symptomatic with moodiness, inability to concentrate, hot flashes, weight gain, or fatigue.

5.   Women who have low testosterone and low libido.

6.   Women who have hormone-related migraine headaches.

7.   Women who are suffering from poor short-term memory and loss of multitasking skills.

8.   Women who developed osteopenia or osteoporosis before sixty years old.

9.   Postmenopausal women who want to achieve the best results from hormone replacement therapy to help prevent dementia, osteoporosis, or slow down the aging process.

Breast Cancer and Hormone Therapy

Susan's story—

I am Susan, fifty-nine years old, and a survivor of breast cancer. I was only thirty-eight when I diagnosed with breast cancer. I had a mastectomy; in fact, I had three surgeries in a year and a half. I also went into early menopause during that time. I suppose being reproductive was something that Mother Nature thought was not in my best interest any more. I suffered for a long time without hormone replacement therapy because no doctors wanted to risk my having cancer again. My life became so sad. I could not sleep and lost the ability to have good focus and to concentrate. My doctor told me that I had the hormone levels of a woman in her eighties. This scared me. I looked older than my years. I had osteopenia (loss of bone density that is considered a precursor to osteoporosis) and vaginal atrophy to a serious degree. My husband and I had not been active sexually for over seven years. It was pretty devastating for me.

I became so depressed that I seriously considered suicide. I literally felt every morning like I was pretty much dead anyway. It seemed as if my feet were already in the grave. Then I met a doctor in Arizona, who did the initial recommendation for insertion of pellets. The pellets have changed my life so much. My husband and I are active again. The cellular structure of my skin all over my body and in my vaginal area is much thicker. I am alert and astute. Since I had gone through early menopause and had lost my sex drive, I felt as if I was not a sexy person anymore. But after getting the pellets, I have started taking belly dancing and I feel very sensual and sexual again. This has been a remarkable turnaround.

I am so very lucky to be alive and have this therapy available to me. It took a long time to find a doctor who was willing to give hormone replacement therapy to me.

By maintaining healthy levels of hormones, the body can better deal with cancer cells. It is wonderful to be a happy, vibrant, and productive member of society. Since starting the pellets, I have earned my broker's license and started my own real estate company.

Fifty years ago, one in every twenty women was diagnosed with breast cancer; now it is one in every six or seven. Birth control pills and hormone replacement therapy have been named as the culprits for this dramatic change in statistics. Similarly, consider the rate of prostate cancer in men. It was also one in twenty only fifty years ago and is now one in every five men, just as with women. But men, unlike women, have not been receiving hormone replacement as routinely as women. So, if hormone replacement is the cause for the increase of breast cancer in women, what is the explanation for the increase of prostate cancer in men? Part of the explanation is that both sexes are living appreciably longer, and that these cancers increase in frequency with age. Also both men and women are now being examined more routinely than at any other time and this will increase the number of cancers found. Fifty years ago, there were no such things as mammograms and PSA exams.

Another part of the answer can be found by looking at other factors. First, there are many chemicals and toxins in the environment which people did not have to contend with fifty years ago. Many of these chemicals and toxins are carcinogens (cancer causing) or hormone impostors, which means they are not actually hormones but can stimulate hormone receptors and cause unwanted results in the body. Another factor is that we are so much more stressed today with a fast-paced lifestyle that is inundated by wireless technology, loud music, and nonstop noise. Higher levels of stress lower our immunity. When immunity is reduced, cancer and other illnesses occur at increased rates.

As we discussed in the previous chapter, bio-identical estrogen replacement therapy with pellets, balanced with bio-identical progesterone and testosterone does not increase the breast cancer rate, not even for women already diagnosed with breast cancer after cancer treatment.

Davelaar, who studied 267 women for twenty-five years, found that women using estradiol pellets had less cancer of the breast than a control group that received no hormone treatment.[34]

Most women develop breast cancer when they are menopausal, the premenopausal ones usually become menopausal after chemotherapy or radiation for breast cancer. Many of them suffer tremendously with menopausal symptoms, especially from depression, insomnia, fatigue and low libido. Scared by the possibility of recurrence of breast cancer and warnings from their physicians, they suffer silently without seeking hormone treatment.

This suffering is needless. There is enough scientific evidence that proper hormone treatment improves the quality of life and boosts the immune system, and thus does not increase the likelihood of a recurrence of cancer.

Breast Cancer Prevention

Breast cancer is one of the most common cancers in females. The older you are, the higher the rate of breast cancer. Breast cancer has a lot to do with environmental toxins, especially xenohormones (chemicals that mimic the effect of estrogen and cause DNA mutations).

There are ways to reduce breast cancer:

1. Reduce Exposure to Environmental Toxins — Hormones are injected into animals. Thus the beef, pork and chicken, as well as milk, cheese, and eggs contain the injected hormones. Make sure to buy organic meats and produce to avoid exposure to these xenohormones. Also, reduce your exposure to pesticides, plastics, and other industrial by-products.

2. Improve Detoxification — It is important to detoxify the estrogen in our bodies once it has performed its vital functions, as the longer it stays in the body, the greater the risk it can lead to estrogen dominance or breast

cancer. Once estrogen is detoxified, it can be processed for elimination.

There are several ways to improve estrogen detoxification:

- Diet: Diets high in cruciferous vegetables such as broccoli, cauliflower, cabbage, and sprouts can increase the C-2 hydroxylation pathway.

- Supplements: Intake of nutrients involved in liver Phase I and Phase II detoxification pathways, including vitamins A, B6, B12, C, folate, magnesium, zinc, selenium, glycine, taurine, glutamine, cysteine, and methionine.

- Probiotics: Probiotics, which are healthy intestinal bacteria, can reduce the harmful bacteria that may interfere with estrogen excretion.

- Fiber can improve elimination.

- Evening Primrose Oil, 1000 mg daily, helps to reduce inflammation of the breast tissue.

3. Improve Your Immunity:

   a. Proper nutrition, focus on a diet that reduces inflammation.

   b. Make sleep a priority.

   c. Stress reduction and coping skills.

   d. Regular exercise.

4. Balance Hormones:

   a. Balance estrogen with testosterone and progesterone, if needed.

   b. Optimize good hormones such as melatonin, DHEA, thyroid hormone, and growth hormone (HGH).

   c. Reduce harmful hormones such as insulin and cortisol.

As discussed previously, hormone balance protects the breast cells. These methods not only protect us from breast cancer, they also reduce estrogen dominance related conditions such as fibrocystic breast disease, premenstrual tension, heavy menstrual bleeding, and fibroid tumors.

HRT and Menopausal Women

It is not a given that all menopausal women need bio-identical hormone replacement therapy, but nearly everyone can benefit from it.

If you are menopausal and have good adrenal function, a healthy, stress free lifestyle, no family history of diabetes, hypertension, osteoporosis, senile dementia, and no menopausal symptoms, you may choose not to use any hormone replacement therapy. Remember, bio-identical hormone replacement therapy reduces cardiovascular diseases, Alzheimer's disease, dementia, osteoporosis, and muscle loss.

The misconception is that if your hot flashes are gone, a woman is finished with menopause, whereas in truth starting into menopause is the first step towards aging and dying. The problem is that degenerative diseases such as osteoporosis, memory loss, atherosclerosis, fatigue, decreased immunity, and arthritis do not come all at once; they progress gradually and often imperceptibly until their presence is too painful or obvious to ignore. Keeping sex hormones in the younger age range, combined with a healthy lifestyle, can slow down or prevent these aging related diseases.

As an internist, I have seen many women in their seventies and eighties who had already developed osteoporosis, dementia, urinary incontinence, and cardiovascular diseases. By this time, their conditions have become very difficult to treat. But even at this stage, their quality of life can improve with bio-identical hormone pellet therapy.

Laboratory Testing for Hormones

In order to implant the correct dosage of pellets, the body's baseline hormone levels need to be established. These can be determined by blood tests. Several blood tests are involved in evaluating hormone functions. First and foremost is FSH (follicular stimulating hormone). This hormone is secreted by the pituitary gland in the brain, which is the master regulator of the hormone systems. FSH regulates estrogen. If the body needs estrogen, FSH rises to stimulate the ovaries to produce more estrogen. If the body has enough estrogen, FSH decreases since it does not need to stimulate the ovaries to produce more estrogen.

Before menopause, FSH is typically below ten. After menopause, it is between twenty-five and 120. The higher the FSH, the more the body needs estrogen. Most women do not feel good if their FSH levels are over fifty. At a perimenopausal stage, when women are still having periods, FSH can be unreliable — both high and low —if the samples were obtained at different times because as estrogen declines, the FSH rises, which stimulates the ovaries to produce more estrogen. Then FSH declines, which leads to reduced estrogen. At this stage many women are symptomatic with hot flashes, night sweats, irregular periods, or mood swings due to fluctuations of their hormone levels. Yet if they only examine blood tests, their doctors may well tell them that they are fine, and not menopausal, as some women have hormone deficient symptoms even when their laboratory tests show their hormone levels to be within normal ranges.

Other hormones I check are estradiol, progesterone, and testosterone, both total and free levels. I also check SHBG (sex hormone binding globulin). A higher SHBG indicates that the level of free hormones is lower and symptoms are more likely to occur.

For adrenal function, I check cortisol and DHEA-S (hormones secreted by adrenal glands) in the morning. The blood tests for adrenal functions are not that reliable and need to be interpreted with the patient's symptoms. If I see that cortisol is very high or very low, it confirms my diagnosis of adrenal stress or exhaustion. Most of the time, I see normal cortisol and low DHEA, which indicates that the patient is in some degree of adrenal fatigue. At this stage, the adrenal glands are still functioning, but the production of DHEA has been lowered to conserve the adrenal glands.

I also check thyroid functions by monitoring TSH, free T3, and free T4. I always check thyroid hormones and adrenal hormones because they are so intimately related to sex hormones. Just like an orchestra, many musicians are involved and they have to perform harmoniously. With hormone replacement therapy, we need to pay attention to all the hormones, especially the major players of the sex, adrenal, and thyroid hormones as people feel their best and will be their healthiest when their hormones are balanced.

Side Effects of Pellets Therapy

Side effects of pellet therapy are few, and at best rare, if done by well trained and experienced physicians. The insertion procedure, on occasion, may cause the possibility of slight pain, bleeding, and infection of the incision site. There may be transient breast tenderness and water retention (ankle swelling) that disappears quickly and usually only occurs with the first insertion.

The real issue is proper dosage of hormone pellets. If the dosage is too low, a person will not feel much improvement. If the dosage is too high, there may be side effects. For instance, if estradiol is too high a woman can develop breast soreness, retain water, or gain fat. If testosterone is too high, individuals can become more aggressive or preoccupied with sexual thoughts; and acne or facial hair can develop. This may also lead to male pattern baldness in the long term. Again, this is where we advise you see a well trained and experienced physician.

Another problem is spotting or menstruation, which is usually the result of insufficient progesterone to balance estrogen's growth effect on the lining of the uterus. This most commonly occurs because a patient does not take progesterone correctly. It can also be due to fibroid tumors, endometrial polyps, and in rare instances, endometrial cancer. If bleeding persists after increasing the dosage of progesterone, a pelvic ultrasound is required, along with an endometrial biopsy.

It is a good idea to start conservatively when it comes to pellet dosage. It is easy to add more pellets, but it is very difficult to remove the pellets after implantation. The pellet dosage also needs to be adjusted periodically according to each individual's response to achieve optimal results.

Contraindications for Pellet Therapy

There are certain conditions that must be considered when determining if pellet therapy is suitable for someone. It is not advisable to give pellet therapy to persons with the following conditions.

1. Untreated breast, uterine or ovarian cancer. For women who have finished their breast cancer treatment and exhibit no evidence of residual cancer, I do offer testosterone, with or without a very small dose of estradiol, if they want to receive pellet therapy. This also applies to women who have had their uterus or ovaries removed due to cancer and who exhibit no evidence of residual cancer. I will not administer treatment if the patient or I have any doubts.

2. History of fibroid tumors. Since estrogen may cause growth of fibroids, estrogen doses have to be modified to a lower level to prevent bleeding. I recommend that women who have large fibroids have them treated first by surgery or uterine artery embolization before starting therapy.

3. History of multiple chemical sensitivities or Leaky Gut Syndrome can have adverse effects due to a toxin overload. In these cases I need to detoxify these patients first and treat gut issues, if there are any. Once this is accomplished we can begin using pellet therapy, although more cautiously and with reduced dosage.

Self-assessment for Estrogen Dominance and PMS

Considering their importance to our health and well-being, it is crucial that our hormones exist in a state of balance. To help gauge your current state of hormonal balance, take a moment to consider the following questions.

1. Do you have heavy menstrual bleeding?

2. Do you have breast tenderness before your period?

3. Do you have fibrocystic breast disease or a uterine fibroid tumor?

4. Do you have mood swings, anxiety, or depression before your period?

5. Do you have water retention or do you feel bloated?

6. Do you have migraine headaches associated with your menstrual cycle?

If you answered "yes" to more than one question, you may have estrogen dominance, which is an imbalance between estrogen and progesterone.

Self-assessment for Testosterone Deficiency

As we have seen, testosterone also plays a very important role in women's health. Consider the following questions to gain a better idea of where your levels of testosterone currently stand.

1. Do you have low libido?

2. Do you experience mental fogginess or have difficulty concentrating?

3. Do you feel depressed or anxious?

4. Do you feel fatigued or lack interest in doing things?

5. Are you losing muscle tone or is it hard to build muscle mass even with exercise?

6. Are you gaining fat in your abdominal area?

7. Do you have dry skin?

8. Are you experiencing vaginal dryness?

9. Do you have migraine headaches?

If you answered "yes" to more than two questions, you may have testosterone deficiency.

Points to Remember

1. Bio-identical hormone replacement therapy, if done right, does not increase the risk of breast cancer.

2. Subcutaneously (under the skin), implanted hormones in the pellet form, is the most physiological route of delivery, and they achieve the best results in terms of minimizing menopausal symptoms.

3. It is important to replace and balance deficient sex hormones because the benefits go beyond reducing menopausal symptoms. Proper hormone balance actually prevents age related diseases and slows down the aging process.

4. Hormone replacement therapy has to be individualized and monitored to achieve the best results and to reduce or eliminate side effects.

5. Testosterone deficiency in women is a neglected problem that can occur even in young women.

6. Adrenal fatigue is very common. Menopause makes adrenal fatigue worse and vice versa.

7. Thyroid, adrenal, and sex hormones are interrelated. Replacing one can affect the others. They must all be monitored and treated together, as needed, to stay in harmonious balance and optimize optimal health.

Chapter 5

Male Testosterone Deficiency

There is no doubt hormones play a significant role in women's health. The life enhancing benefits of bio-identical hormone therapy that were discussed last chapter: physical vitality, emotional balance, disease prevention, and the slowing down of the aging process continue to be documented by medical studies and confirmed by the patient success stories we witness in our practices every day. But did you know that men can also stand to benefit greatly from bio-identical hormone therapy? This is true. More men than ever are becoming aware of the detrimental effects of hormone loss on their bodies and the potential of pellet therapy to restore their former robustness and zest for life. While it is true that hormones like testosterone exist in much higher amounts in men, the gradual decline of this vital hormone causes just as many problems for men as the loss of estrogen does in women. For instance, take my patient Lee and the many difficulties he faced when his levels of testosterone declined dangerously low.

Lee's story—

I am Lee, aged sixty-three. A decade ago I was CEO of a public health care company when a hereditary iron metabolism disease, hemochromatosis, forced my retirement. With iron poisoned organs, my convalescence took years. Dedicated exercise helped, but I was hampered with vital organ scar tissue, and I was forced into having a pint of blood drained every two months for the rest of my life to remove excess iron build-up. Since my testicles were damaged and my libido had suffered, I asked my doctor for testosterone injections. Even though my blood levels were very low, he declined, saying that it was just something I would have to live with. So, I did. Year upon year out of unnecessary necessity, I wrote off most of my sex life. What a void. What a waste. What a tragedy. Totally unnecessary!

Then, I heard about bio-identical hormone replacement therapy, which led me to a highly trained, board certified internal medicine specialist, Karen Sun, M.D., in Irvine, California. She was wonderful, a real and totally dedicated doctor who immediately seized upon my chronic panoply of male hormone-deficient symptoms of fatigue, insomnia, anxiety, depression, "feeling old," and, of course, a minimal sex drive. Fresh blood tests proved that my free testosterone levels were next to zero. Dr. Sun quickly initiated just under the skin hormone replacement pellets, a painless, fifteen minute procedure. She closely monitored my astonishing rebirth thereafter.

Within weeks I felt ten, maybe twenty years younger. I slept well and, at long last, woke up every morning refreshed and free of cobwebs. I acquired zest, which lasted all day. My anxiety and depression dissipated, and I became hungry for love. Although the hormones increased my appetite, I thwarted weight gain by increasing my exercise, which I suddenly had the energy to accomplish.

Testosterone has been used successfully for years to treat men with abnormally low testosterone levels, a medical condition called male hypogonadism. In most men, testosterone secretion starts to decline at the rate of 1 to 3 percent a year after age thirty. This means that by age fifty, a man may have lost 20 to 60 percent of his testosterone production. By the age of seventy, 70 percent of all men fit into the criteria of hypogonadism. The marked decline in energy levels, mental focus, libido, and emotional stability that accompanies this process has become so common and widespread that a new term, "andropause," has been coined to describe the transition men undergo when hormone levels bottom out.

Andropause, like menopause, is due to the decline of testosterone but, unlike women who experience a sudden drop of hormones, it occurs gradually and the symptoms are less dramatic.

Symptoms of Andropause and Testosterone Deficiency

- Decreased energy and fatigue
- Reduced muscle strength and mass, less exercise endurance, and prolonged recovery from exercise
- Decreased cognitive function, such as poor memory or lack of mental sharpness
- Less sexual interest and/or performance
- Loss of interest; crabby, depressed mood
- Weight gain
- Insomnia, decreased quality of sleep
- Thinning of body hair and dry brittle hair
- Joint pain
- Osteoporosis or decreased bone density (X-ray finding)

Diagnosis of Testosterone Deficiency

1. Blood test for both total and free testosterone level:

    a. Most testosterone binds with SHBG (sex hormone binding globulin) and is not active. Like a car in a car carrier, it's not driving on the road. Only free testosterone, testosterone that is not bound with SHBG, is small enough to enter the body's cells and work. The production of total testosterone decreases with age, but the SHBG remains the same. This leads to a reduced amount of free testosterone and consequently of the functions testosterone provides. To determine the amount of testosterone available to perform in the body, it is important to check both total testosterone and free testosterone.

2.   Blood test for estradiol level:

   a.   Aging also causes a testosterone-estrogen imbalance in men. Specifically, reduced free testosterone with the same or increased estrogen changes the ratio of testosterone to estrogen. A testosterone-estrogen imbalance can cause many diseases associated with aging, including heart attack, stroke, and prostate hypertrophy (enlargement).

Common Reasons for Testosterone-estrogen Imbalance

- Liver dysfunction.
  - o   As the body's major detoxification organ, the liver eliminates excess estrogen and sex hormone-binding protein. The liver can have reduced function due to the effects of alcohol, drugs, infection, heart failure, aging, or liver diseases, which leads to increased estrogen and sex hormone-binding protein.
- Obesity.
  - o   Fat cells, especially around the abdominal area, secrete estrogen and aromatase, which is an enzyme that converts testosterone to estrogen. Increased estrogen in men further increases abdominal fat. This becomes a vicious cycle.
- Nutritional deficiency, especially zinc, which is a natural aromatase inhibitor, will make things worse by turning more testosterone into unwanted estrogen.

Testosterone and the Prostate Gland

Many people, including doctors, think prostate cancer is linked to testosterone. This is the most common reason that men shy away from testosterone replacement therapy. Most published scientific papers, however, suggest otherwise.[42,43] Estrogens, especially the environmental xenohormones, not testosterone, are more to blame.

Living longer contributes to the increase in the incidence of cancers, especially prostate cancer. Additionally, fifty years ago there were not as many chemicals and toxins in the environment to disrupt the body's hormone systems. Now we have so many more toxins, especially xenoestrogens, from certain foods, pesticides and plastics. These are aggravating factors that I see contributing to the cause of the increase of cancers in the reproductive systems of both men and women.

If prostate cancer cells are present, however, increasing the level of testosterone will speed the growth of cancer. This is why the PSA (prostate specific antigen) blood level should be checked before and after testosterone treatment.

For men who have prostate hypertrophy (enlargement), testosterone treatment can increase the size of the prostate even more by its conversion to DHT (dihydrotestoster-one) and estradiol, both of which can stimulate prostate growth. Proscar (a prescription medicine) reduces DHT and Aromasin (a prescription medicine) is an aromatase inhibitor that can reduce the conversion of testosterone to estrogen. Both medications can be used to prevent or slow down prostate growth.

Saw palmetto is a supplement that can reduce DHT formation. It also inhibits the binding of estrogen to prostate cells and the binding of DHT to the prostate gland. Saw palmetto reduces inflammation of the prostate and relaxes the sphincter tone around the urethra so the flow of urine can improve. For these reasons, saw palmetto has become a very popular prostate supplement for men. Another popular supplement is chrysin, which is derived from the plant Passiflora caerulea. It works as a natural aromatase inhibitor. It is also a potent antioxidant and has the added benefit of reducing inflammation. Formulas that combine all the protective herbal agents, such as saw palmetto, lycopene, chrysin, and zinc are recommended for prostate health.

Testosterone and Depression

Have you ever encountered a grumpy old man? You do not have to grow old to be grumpy, but there certainly are a lot of grumpy men who are old. There is a hormonal reason for that too.

Published studies show that HRT increases the sense of well-being in andropausal men.[44] Studies also show that a low level of testosterone is associated with anxiety, depression, irritability and other psychological disorders in andropausal men. An article in the *American Journal of Geriatric Psychiatry* reviewed studies published from 1966 to 1999 to determine if there was a moderate decline of total testosterone and, more significantly, a decline of bioavailable (free) testosterone in aging males.[45] The article's survey revealed some interesting findings. Elderly males who were depressed appeared to have the lowest testosterone levels. In males with normal testosterone levels, HRT did not have a significant effect on mood. However, in treating depressed men with low testosterone levels, HRT was shown to be very effective. This article advocated HRT as a primary or adjunct treatment of depression in elderly males. Another article showed that testosterone replacement therapy is more effective than antidepressants in men with lower testosterone levels.[46]

Testosterone and the Cardiovascular System

A recent study published in the *Journal of American College of Cardiology* shows that testosterone helps to protect men from atherosclerosis (hardening of the arteries).[47]

They performed ultrasound testing on aging men to assess the thickness of the carotid artery, the artery that supplies blood to the brain. As the testosterone level dropped, the artery wall thickness increased, which impaired delivery of oxygen to the brain thus leading to dementia and stroke.

Testosterone helps to build muscles, including heart muscles.[48] Testosterone also dilates coronary arteries, reduces heart attacks, reduces high blood pressure, and helps to lower cholesterol levels.[49,50]

Testosterone causes erection by dilating blood vessels in the penis due to stimulating the production of nitrous oxide. The same effect also happens in coronary arteries. The most abundant receptor sites found for testosterone are not in the penis or the brain, but are located in the coronary blood vessels.

If you have high blood pressure or cardiovascular disease, you should check your free testosterone and estrogen levels.

Treating testosterone deficiency and improving the testosterone/estrogen ratio may be one of the most effective and natural ways to treat cardiovascular diseases.

Testosterone and Insulin — Diabetes

Stephen's story —

I am Stephen, I am in my mid-fifties. I had been a very healthy, energetic, active business professional until in my early forties, when I started feeling somewhat off. My weight gradually increased by twenty pounds, which was somewhat disconcerting. I just didn't feel right. Then, after I visited a marshmallow factory in Las Vegas and tried some samples, I started to feel terrible on the drive back to California. Normally, I could drive long distances with no problem. But on this drive, I didn't even make it to the state line. I had to ask my wife, Debby, to drive. That had never happened before. Then I passed out and woke up hours later in Newport Beach. It turns out that I was in a diabetic coma. That was the cornerstone of my health problems, which led to my seeing a very reputable internist.

Every time I mentioned a problem to my internist, he gave me a prescription for it. But I was feeling worse as the years went by. Indeed, the more medicine he gave me, the worse I felt. And, always, my doctor's answer to my every health question was: "Well, you are getting older. You're going to have some pain with one thing or another." None of this made sense to me. So, I started asking around and doing research. That is when I learned about hormones in general, and specifically, as a guy I was focusing on testosterone. I asked my internist about my testosterone levels and just got his typical answer about getting older. Then he gave me another prescription for something completely unrelated.

I pushed my internist to test my testosterone level. A man's testosterone should be at 1,000; mine was ninety-three. A couple of things don't work well at a T level of ninety-three. Not only that, the little blue pill (Viagra) did not work for me and that really concerned me. So, I went on a mission to learn everything I could about hormone replacement. I have followed Suzanne Somers and her books on the subject.

Then, I found Karen Sun, M.D. through a couple who are friends of ours. At a dinner at their home, I noticed that the wife had more energy than usual, and I asked if she happened to be on bio-identical hormones, not a typical conversation for us. But I had been doing research and thought I would discuss it with her. She confirmed that was true and then explained how Dr. Sun had done the procedure to implant pellets about the size of grains of rice. She added that her general overall feeling was now just fantastic. I told her, "You are a sign from heaven."

So, I went to see Dr. Sun and she spent more time counseling me in our first session than the years of visits I had spent with my internist, collectively. She took blood tests and gave me information my other doctor never talked about with me. She also told me that she thought we could get me off most of the medications I was taking. Two days after she gave me the pellets I felt like I was in my early thirties again. Within five days, every ache in my body was gone.

Since I have been on the pellets, I have lost nearly thirty pounds, and that is without doing anything special to lose weight. I just feel great now, and we have managed to eliminate most of my meds. Also, emotionally I had been experiencing a high level of edginess and things would set me off more quickly before I was on the pellets. I was not quite as patient, but with the pellets, my emotions are very much in check. I am a touchy- feely type of person, and when the romantic part of my life dropped to almost zero, I was not happy. I did not want to hang up that saddle for the rest of my life. Ever since I've been pelletized, that area has come roaring back. I feel great!

Studies have linked low levels of testosterone with diabetes.[51,52] Testosterone replacement therapy reduces insulin resistance. Dhindsa et al. showed that a third of men with type II diabetes have low free testosterone levels.[53] A low level of testosterone causes low lean muscle mass and higher abdominal fat, which leads to insulin resistance and increased risk for cardiovascular diseases. Testosterone replacement reduces body fat, increases lean muscle, and improves strength. Many diabetic men who have low testosterone suffer from depression, poor memory, insomnia, fatigue, low bone density, heart disease, and erectile dysfunction. In Steven's case, he was able to lose weight, lower his blood pressure and diabetic medication after the pellet treatment. Most importantly, his life is back!

Testosterone therapy should be incorporated into treatment plans for diabetic patients with low testosterone levels and may well be one of the most effective and natural treatments available.

Testosterone and Alzheimer's Disease

Research is revealing a strong link between low testosterone levels and Alzheimer's disease. One study shows that longitudinal assessment of serum free testosterone concentration predicts memory performance and cognitive status in elderly men.[54] Another study also supports that testosterone replacement reduces the risk of Alzheimer's disease by preventing the production of beta-amyloid protein.[55]

In my practice, I routinely observe that mood and mental sharpness in patients improve after testosterone replacement therapy. This is the most common reason my patients want to continue the treatment. They not only appreciate the benefits of an improved libido, they also welcome the mental sharpness and enhanced sense of well-being that accompanies testosterone therapy. Indeed testosterone replacement therapy is one of the most important preventive methods for dementia and Alzheimer's disease.

Testosterone and Osteoporosis

According to the National Osteoporosis Foundation, two million men in the U.S. have osteoporosis and another three million are at risk. Gradual decline of testosterone (T) is the most common reason for osteoporosis in aging men. In one study, 59 percent of men with hip fractures had low T, compared with 18 percent of men in the control group.[56] Fractures occur at a later age in men than in women because men's bones are denser than women's. Testosterone receptors are present in osteoblasts (bone-forming cells), and many studies report the beneficial effects of testosterone treatment in older men, showing an increase in bone mineral density and a slowing of bone degeneration.

For men affected by osteoporosis, getting testosterone replacement therapy may work better than taking prescription medications, with the added plus of providing a wide spectrum of benefits such as enhanced energy, emotional balance, mental clarity, and revitalized libido.

Is Testosterone Replacement Therapy the Answer for Aging Men?

Do you want to increase your muscle mass, strengthen your bones, improve your cardiovascular system, boost your mood, sharpen your memory, charge up your libido, and improve your energy? Does anyone ever say "no" to this? Of course not! To men suffering from the ill-effects of hormone loss and age-related diseases, these things may very well sound like key ingredients to the fountain of youth.

Yet far from being a fantasy, treatment with bio-identical testosterone pellets can be a very real part of men's lives, bringing benefits that enhance the quality of their lives tremendously. According to the statistics, men everywhere are standing up and taking notice. HRT in aging men is growing in popularity. According to IMS Health, a company that tracks pharmaceutical sales, 2.4 million testosterone prescriptions were filled in 2004, more than twice the amount that were filled in 2000. The questions arise: Is testosterone safe? What is the down side? What is the best delivery method? So far, no long-term human study has been done, but we can borrow what we have learned from hormone replacement therapy for women. In general, the rules should be the same.

Testosterone — Routes of Delivery

1. Intramuscular Injection

    a. An intramuscular injection is given every two weeks and results in fluctuating hormone levels. It can be very high in the first few days then drop down quickly. It is a hormone roller coaster! Also, the drugs available for injections are not bio-identical testosterone; Depo-Testosterone (testosterone cypionate) and methyltestosterone are commonly used.

2. Transdermal: Patch, Cream, or Gel

    a. Androderm patch is available by prescription. The patch needs to be changed daily and skin irritation can be a problem. AndroGel is also available by prescription. The gel or cream can be rubbed into the skin on the lower abdomen, upper arm, or shoulder area. It causes less skin irritation than the patch. Users must avoid showering or bathing for several hours after application to ensure adequate absorption. A potential side effect is the possibility of transferring the testosterone to your partner. The absorption rate may vary resulting in an insignificant improvement of the testosterone level, and that is why many men treated with this route do not feel significant improvement.

3. Oral

    a. The oral form of delivery is not a recommended route. Due to processing through the liver, taking testosterone orally may cause an unfavorable cholesterol profile, and an increase in the risk of blood clots along with possible liver damage.

4. Sublingual (under the tongue)

    a. The sublingual route allows the testosterone to be absorbed directly into the bloodstream. It becomes oral;

however, if it is swallowed before it dissolves and is absorbed. It can also cause gum irritation and may have an unpleasant taste. The sublingual route causes a surge of testosterone, which lasts ten to twelve hours, and it needs to be used twice a day.

5.   Pellet Implants

a.   Bio-identical hormones pellet implants are placed subcutaneously just under the skin. These hormones are released into the bloodstream slowly and last between four to six months. Since it bypasses the liver, this is by far the most physiological and effective delivery system of the right hormones in the proper dosage that attains a steady blood level all of the time.

In my practice, I have seen many men who have tried testosterone in the form of gels, patches or shots, but did not achieve the results they wanted, whereas subcutaneously implanted pellets have worked well for them. Plus, pellets are a very easy system of administration. There is no gel, cream, or patch to apply every day; just a simple procedure performed every four to six months.

Rules of Testosterone Replacement

Just as with women's hormone replacement, there are special rules to observe when utilizing testosterone therapy in men.

1.   Only replace testosterone when it is at a low functional level for that patient.

2.   Use bio-identical hormones.

3.   Monitor the hormone levels; be sure they are in a normal range and maintain a proper testosterone to estrogen ratio.

4.   Use the most physiological route of delivery, which is either transdermal, sublingual, or subcutaneous pellet implants.

5.   Regularly monitor the PSA and estrogen level to make sure it does not increase with the hormone treatment.

Indications for Testosterone Replacement

The following symptoms may indicate that your testosterone levels are low.

- Depression, crabby mood, or loss of interest in activities
- Fatigue or low energy level
- Low libido or erectile dysfunction
- Poor memory, lack of concentration
- Reduced muscle mass
- Osteoporosis or osteopenia
- Diabetes, hypertension, and cardiovascular diseases Insomnia or poor quality of sleep
- Weight gain, especially fat around the middle

Side Effects of Testosterone Replacement

When considering the possibility of side effects in testosterone replacement therapy, it is important to remember that the side effects of HRT are related to super high dosages. The side effects do not happen if it is done with physiological dosage and blood tests are done regularly. These common side effects are: increase bone marrow production of red blood cells, which leads to an increase in blood volume and blood pressure, and an increased risk of blood clots and may cause acne, and lead to testicular shrinkage (atrophy), increased prostate hypertrophy and male pattern baldness.

Contraindications for Testosterone Replacement

There are instances when testosterone replacement therapy should not be considered. Do not use when there is either:

1. Untreated prostate cancer or breast cancer (rare but can occur in men).
2. Untreated benign prostate hypertrophy (BPH).

Points to Remember

1. Testosterone production declines with age. By the age of seventy, 70 percent of men have testosterone deficiency.

2. Testosterone replacement therapy is not solely meant to boost the libido. It improves mood and memory, builds muscle and bone density, reduces body fat, and helps to prevent or treat hypertension, diabetes and cardiovascular diseases associated with testosterone deficiency.

3. Use bio-identical hormones and a physiological route of delivery such as gel, patch or subcutaneously implanted pellets if you decide to do testosterone replacement therapy. Pellet implants are the easiest and most effective treatment method. Consider trying pellet therapy if use of the patch, cream, or gel does not produce the results you desire.

4. Patients' free and total testosterone levels should always be monitored: higher than normal hormone levels may lead to side effects and complications.

5. PSA levels should be monitored closely, especially in the first year of receiving testosterone treatment.

6. It is also important to monitor estradiol levels and the testosterone-to-estradiol ratio. The use of an aromatase inhibitor should be considered if estradiol is too high.

7. Nutritional supplements with antioxidants, minerals, vitamins C and E, lycopene, zinc, selenium, and herbs such as saw palmetto and chrysin are helpful for prostate health.

Chapter 6

Adrenal Fatigue — The Stress Epidemic

The adrenal glands secrete hormones to help the body cope with stress. About the size of a walnut, the adrenal glands sit on top of the kidneys and produce powerful hormones to sustain the body and its life processes. As a matter of fact, we would die without adrenal hormones.

Stress Factors

Stress assaults us every day. Relationships can be stressful due to, among other things, marital problems and divorce, death or illness of family members, or challenges with raising children. Our professional commitments involve such stressors as the need to work long hours, the hassles of commuting, troubles with co-workers, the pressures of deadlines and disliking current employment, being laid off or needing to change jobs. When there is not enough money to pay the bills, the worry created can be quite traumatic. Additionally, we can stress ourselves internally when we worry too much or strive too hard to be perfect.

We can have physical stressors, too, such as surgery, colds or flu, chronic insomnia, injuries, etc. Toxic chemicals in our environment and pollutants in the air also cause inflammation of our bodies and damage our adrenal glands. Chronic stress places a strain on our adrenal glands to over produce stress hormones, which over time leads to adrenal burn out, so called adrenal fatigue.

Adrenal Hormones and Their Actions

Adrenal Medulla — The adrenal medulla (inside part) secretes:

1. Epinephrine (adrenaline).
2. Norepinephrine.

These hormones trigger the body's response to the arousal to "fight or flight." They work on our autonomic (or automatic) nervous system, which increases our blood pressure and heart rate. They also cause muscle contractions.

In the GI (gastrointestinal) system, these hormones cause diarrhea or constipation, which, if chronic, can lead to irritable bowel syndrome. These hormones are also neurotransmitters that stimulate the brain. They put us on high alert if danger threatens. These are also the hormones that give us stage fright.

Adrenal Cortex — The adrenal cortex (outside part) produces several hormones:

1. DHEA and pregnenolone, the precursors to progesterone, testosterone, and estrogen.
2. Cortisol (cortisone), which increases blood sugar. When early humans saw a predator ready to attack, they had to react right away in order to survive. The adrenal glands pump cortisol to increase the blood sugar as the source of energy for the body's ability to respond to extraordinary circumstances. Cortisol also increase adrenaline levels, regulates our immune response, and reduces inflammation.
3. Aldosterone, a hormone that increases body fluids. It increases sodium retention and potassium excretion, leading to fluid retention and increased blood pressure.

Stages of Stress and Adrenal Fatigue

Stress wears down the adrenal glands over time. Hence, damage to the adrenals occurs gradually. The onset of adrenal fatigue is not sudden; rather, it occurs in three stages.

First Stage Adrenal Stress —

The first stage is termed arousal and is referred to as adrenal hyper function. For example, if a person sees a house on fire, the adrenal glands release a spurt of adrenaline, which causes higher blood pressure, rapid heartbeat, greater alertness and more tense muscles. A slower surge of cortisol produces extra blood sugar so that individual can use the energy boost for the fight-or-flight response. When the emergency is gone, the body returns to normal.

Second Stage Adrenal Stress —

The second stage of adrenal stress is called adaptation. Being in a chronically stressed environment is like living in a war zone. A person is prepared to fight at any time and, accordingly, sustains high levels of adrenal hormones that can change the body in several ways:

- Glucose (blood sugar) metabolism is harmfully altered. Elevated levels of cortisol increase blood sugar as a source of energy. If the body does not burn this sugar off, it will store the excess as fat. Higher sugar levels also stimulate insulin secretion from the pancreas. Eventually, chronic elevated cortisol levels lead to weight gain and diabetes.

- The cardiovascular system is negatively impacted. Aldosterone by altering the sodium and potassium ratio increases blood volume and elevates blood pressure. Adrenaline also cause increase heart rate, which is palpitation, and constriction of blood vessel which increases blood pressure in the long run.

- A high cortisol level reduces the transformation of thyroid hormone from T4 to the more active form of T3. This leads to subclinical hypothyroidism, which causes fatigue and further weight gain.

- High cortisol levels can affect our brain function negatively, impairing our memory, inducing brain fog. High adrenaline levels cause anxiety. Combined together, it makes tasks harder to handle.

- Reduced sex hormone production. Stress forces the adrenal glands to produce more stress hormones. The exhausted adrenals produce less DHEA, the precursor of sex hormones. Before menopause, 30 percent of the sex hormones are generated by the adrenal glands and 70 percent by the ovaries. After menopause, the ratio reverses. Most of the sex hormones then must come from the adrenal glands, and if the overworked adrenals are burned out, the body will have a hard time dealing with menopausal symptoms.

- The quality of sleep diminishes. Adrenaline is a neurotransmitter that stimulates the brain. If a person is under stress with too much adrenaline, the brain is overactive at bedtime, and it is hard to relax and fall asleep. Even if people can fall into sleep due to fatigue, they have restless sleep waking up frequently. Poor sleep leads to fatigue, poor memory, and irritability.

- Excessive adrenaline increases muscle contractions, which leads to neck and back pain, as well as tension headaches. Poor sleep further reduces the muscles' ability to rest and relax. Stress has much to do with fibromyalgia, which has two major characteristics: muscle pain all over and insomnia.

- With adrenal fatigue, the immune system also becomes compromised, which leads to more frequent colds and flu. Furthermore, it becomes increasingly difficult to bounce back from illness. Lower immunity also makes individuals more prone to other diseases, including cancer.

At this second stage, a person can still function in high gear, but fatigue starts to set in more often, and many people need to drink coffee or other stimulants to keep going. Weight gain is common, as are diseases such as hypertension, heart attacks, diabetes, fibromyalgia, hypothyroidism, depression, and anxiety.

Third Stage Adrenal Stress —

The third stage of adrenal stress is exhaustion. This is the final stage when people become very fatigued and have difficulty functioning at all. Blood pressure can become low due to low aldosterone, cortisol, and adrenaline. People can feel dizzy especially when suddenly standing or bending over. Recovery from this stage is a long, slow process of equal parts medical treatment and a commitment to lifestyle changes that reduce stressors.

Symptoms of Adrenal Exhaustion

- Difficulty getting up in the morning
- Continuous fatigue not relieved by sleep
- Craving for salt or salty food
- Increased effort to do everyday tasks
- Decreased sex drive
- Decreased ability to handle stress (anxiety)
- Light-headed or dizziness when standing up
- Difficulty recovering from illness or injury
- Depression
- Need to drink coffee or caffeinated soft drinks for energy.
- Brain fog, not being able to concentrate
- Memory loss
- Irritability
- Inability to sleep through the night

Frequently, patients with adrenal fatigue are also carrying diagnosis of chronic fatigue syndrome, fibromyalgia, irritable bowel syndrome, hypothyroidism, chronic insomnia, diabetes, leaky gut syndrome, anxiety, or depression.

Diagnosis and Tests for Adrenal Fatigue

It is hard to diagnose adrenal fatigue until its late stage. One reason is the lack of adequate tests. Another is that the symptoms are insidious and overlap with other diseases. But there are several ways to examine the body for this condition:

1.   The iris cannot hold contraction when light is shined onto the eye. Normally when we shine a light onto one eye, the iris reacts with contraction of the pupil (making it small) and the pupil remains contracted. In adrenal fatigue, the pupil will not be able to hold its contraction and will dilate despite the light still shining on it. This will take place within two minutes and will last from thirty to forty-five seconds before it recovers and contracts again. Sometimes, the iris will contract initially, then dilate, then contract, then dilate again. This inability of the iris to remain contracted occurs in moderate to severe adrenal fatigue, but may not be evident in mild adrenal fatigue. This test is also a good way to determine if an individual has recovered from adrenal fatigue.

2.   Saliva and blood hormone testing. The adrenal hormone levels fluctuate at different times throughout the day. Ideally, levels should be measured four times a day: within one hour of waking, usually from 6:00 to 8:00 a.m., when the levels are highest; then between 11:00 a.m. to 12:00 p.m., again at 4:00 p.m. to 6:00 p.m., followed by one from 10:00 p.m. to 12:00 a.m. Stress levels during the day can affect hormone levels. The blood test measures hormones circulating in the bloodstream. The saliva test reflects tissue hormone levels. We need to check the cortisol and DHEA levels four times a day, so the saliva test is used due to its convenience.

Treatment of Adrenal Fatigue

It takes a long time and dedicated effort to recover from adrenal fatigue. In order for the adrenal glands to be restored to optimal levels of functioning several lifestyle changes are necessary.

Make Sleep a Priority — Sleep is very important for adrenal recovery. For people who have adrenal fatigue, it is best to fall asleep before 10:00 p.m., because the second wind of adrenal hormone secretion hits around 11:00 p.m. If you ride on the second wind, which makes you more energetic and prone to stay up until 1:00 a.m. to 2:00 a.m., you will further exhaust your adrenal glands. Also, not getting up until 8:30 a.m. or 9:00 a.m. helps. This is when the adrenals secrete hormones again; sleeping at this time can be remarkably refreshing.

Steps to help you sleep better:

1. Avoid stimulants such as coffee, tea (except herbal tea), chocolate, or caffeinated soft drinks, especially after noontime.

2. Avoid nighttime tension such as fighting with your spouse or children, watching violent movies or television, paying bills, working at the computer, etc.

3. Make your bedroom comfortable without light or noise stimulation. Also make sure it is well ventilated, not too hot or too cold. Make sure the mattress is comfortable.

4. Wear earplugs if your partner snores.

5. Have a sleep routine such as one hour before you sleep, write a daily review or emotional diary. Ask yourself how you feel emotionally. If there is anything that bothers you, write it down, and ask yourself what you can do to handle it. Then ask yourself to release the negative emotions, be it anger or worry. Also write down what you need to do tomorrow and prioritize it. Afterward, do relaxation exercises such as yoga or Pilates, followed by meditation, which slows down the brain waves and leads to sleep.

6. Take supplements like 400-500 mg magnesium at bedtime, which helps relax the muscles for achieving a deeper sleep; and 1-3 mg melatonin sublingually (under the tongue), which helps to normalize sleep patterns.

7. Other supplements, such as 500-1000 mg tryptophan or 50-100 mg 5-HTP (5- hydroxytryptophan) at night to increase the level of serotonin, which also helps with sleep. Several herbs, such as hops, passion flower, valerian and licorice, also can help. Hypothalamus extract and adrenal extracts both assist in normalizing sleep patterns.

Take Control of Your Diet — The Adrenal Recovery Diet

1. Reduce high glycemic carbohydrates, which can trigger insulin secretion and leads to hypoglycemia and fatigue later. Small, frequent meals help to avoid low blood sugar (hypoglycemia).
2. More salty food is preferable in cases of hypotension (low blood pressure) and dizziness.
3. Breakfast is the most important meal of the day. Plan to eat breakfast every morning.
4. Increase dietary fiber. Using flaxseed meal or psyllium fiber in a smoothie or drink in the morning will help maintain glycemic control, and prevent fatigue in the afternoon.
5. Most people feel fatigued by 4:00 p.m. when the sugar gets low. Eat a nutritious protein snack with hot herbal tea and sit down to take a break.
6. Limit caffeine, alcohol, fried foods, and sweets.
7. Reduce inflammation by reducing processed and refined food with trans fats.
8. Eat a lot of vegetables with different colors. They are rich in antioxidants, and they reduce inflammation. These foods will feed the body with balanced nutrients, including vitamins, minerals, fibers, and electrolytes.
9. Eat nuts and seeds as sources of essential fatty acids, which also reduce inflammation.

Reduce Your Stress

1. Simplify your life, set priorities for what you will dedicate your time and precious energy to accomplish. Do not feel guilty if you are not perfect.
2. Journal your moods and emotions each day, and release negative emotions. Focus on positive thoughts which will change your mood from anxiety, worry, anger, or frustration to joy and happiness. Those feel good emotions will reduce

the stress hormone secretion. Also write down what you need to do the next day; being organized reduces stress.

3. Exercise regularly, particularly relaxation exercises such as yoga or Pilates, which you can do even when you are tired. Stretching exercises help to relax the muscles and reduce muscle spasms and pain.

4. Deep breathing is one of the easiest, yet most effective ways to relax. Studies show breathing five to six times per minute relaxes our body quickly and effectively. Combined with the visualization of peaceful settings, deep breathing can do wonders for the body.

5. Meditation. Picture a cup filled with water and sand. Shake the cup and the water becomes murky. But let the cup sit for a while and the sand settles down at the bottom of the cup and the water becomes clear again. Meditation helps the mind to become clear. While meditating, let thoughts come through you and do not dwell on any particular thought, just let them pass through. Gradually, the mind will calm itself and thoughts will become less frequent, as the brain waves become slower. You can use meditation before sleep if you have a hard time falling to sleep.

6. Find things you enjoy doing and do them regularly. Simple things such as taking a walk along the beach, listening to your favorite music, gardening, dancing, a nice bath or massage, picking flowers, or having lunch with a friend will help you relax and enjoy each day.

7. Do not dwell on the negatives, which have a way of building on themselves and dragging you down. Think positively; appreciate what you have. Gratitude helps keep the focus on the positive aspects of life and assists in responding to life dynamically.

8. Build quiet time into your day. Slow down, take a break, and take deep breaths. Lie down after lunch for a refreshing rest for twenty to thirty minutes will help the energy production in the afternoon and evening.

9. Laughter is the best medicine. Watch comedies, joke with friends, and be silly.

10. Build healthy relationships.

Supplements for Recovery from Adrenal Fatigue

Vitamin C

Vitamin C is the most important of all the vitamins and minerals involved in adrenal metabolism, as it is essential to the manufacturing of adrenal hormones. Vitamin C also increases adrenal function and stimulates the immune function.

The best vitamin C occurs in nature, as this source of vitamin provides the bioflavonoids that enhance its antioxidant effect. Humans do not make vitamin C so it must be derived from food sources, including colored vegetables such as green leafy vegetables and tomatoes, as well as citrus fruits. The highest amount of vitamin C is in the sprouts of any seed and grain. The younger the plant, the more vitamin C it contains.

In the case of adrenal fatigue, vitamin C from food alone may not be sufficient. However, unless you can drink several pounds of fresh juice that you make for yourself daily, it is much simpler to take 500-1,000 mg. of vitamin C with bioflavonoids (at a 2:1 ratio) two to three times a day. Do not stop vitamin C suddenly. Taper it gradually, as you require less as you recover from adrenal fatigue.

Vitamin E

Vitamin E is not directly involved in the metabolism of adrenal hormones, yet it is essential in an indirect way. Manufacturing adrenal hormones creates harmful free radicals, which slow down the enzyme proteins and damage adrenal glands. Vitamin E absorbs and neutralizes free radicals. It takes both vitamins C and E working together to keep the adrenal glands functioning at optimal levels.

It is important to choose the right type of vitamin E. Most vitamin E sold in stores is d-alpha-tocopherol, but the type of vitamin E needed for adrenal regeneration is beta-tocopherol. Taking mixed tocopherols (d-beta, d-gamma, and d-delta) with vitamin E is important. Take 800 IU a day with meals.

B Vitamins

- Pantothenic Acid: One of the B vitamins, pantothenic acid, is essential for the production of energy. The body converts it into acetyl-CoA, a substance that is critical for the conversion of sugar (glucose) into energy in the mitochondria inside the cells and tissues. Adrenal cells need a lot of pantothenic acid because much energy is needed for adrenal hormone production. 1,500 mg per day is recommended.

- Vitamin B6: Vitamin B6 is a helpful cofactor in the manufacturing of hormones by the adrenal glands. Take 50-100 mg a day for moderate to severe adrenal fatigue.

- B Complex: The entire B complex is needed in small quantities throughout the production of adrenal hormones. Food sources of B complex are whole grains, miso, brewer's yeast, liver, and rice bran. When buying B complex, it is important to buy it in the proper proportion of 50-100 mg of B6, 75-125 mg of B3 and 200-400 µg of B12.

Other Supplements

- Magnesium: Magnesium is also involved in energy production, and adrenal recovery depends on the presence of magnesium. Vitamin C, pantothenic acid, magnesium, and others work together for adrenal function.

- Trace Minerals: Trace minerals include zinc, manganese, selenium,

- Fiber: Fiber helps the body eliminate fat-soluble toxins and thus protects and improves adrenal function. Food sources can be obtained from most vegetables, fruits, seeds, and whole grains.

- Herbs: There are a few herbs, called adaptogens, which help the adrenal glands to function better. They include Rhodiola, licorice root, Siberian ginseng, and ashwagandha. These herbs improve energy and the sense of well-being.

- Rhodiola has been used extensively in Russia and Scandinavia as traditional folk medicine to treat fatigue, mental clarity, and memory. Ashwagandha has traditionally been used in Ayurvedic medicine and has been found to have the effect of reducing stress response and rejuvenation of the body. Siberian Ginseng has been used in China for thousands of years to improve memory and for anti-aging.

Adrenal Cell Extract

Adrenal cortical extracts are from the adrenal cortex of bovine (cows). The first recorded use of bovine adrenal extract was in 1918, and it has been commercially available since then. The extract includes adrenal cell contents and nutrients in the form and proportion used by adrenal glands and contains only small amounts of the adrenal hormones themselves. The extract is generally safe and helps to rebuild adrenal glands.

Hormone Treatments

• DHEA and Pregnenolone: DHEA and pregnenolone are bio-identical adrenal hormones. I use them in small doses sublingually a few times a day and find them very useful in helping with energy, memory, and mental clarity.

• Cortisol: Synthetic cortisol became available in 1950 and has somewhat replaced the use of adrenal cell extract. It is more effective and creates dramatic improvement. However, the down side is that long-term use can suppress our own adrenal function instead of helping adrenal recovery if a high dose is used. For this reason, cortisol should be used only in cases of severe adrenal fatigue and taken only in appropriate physiological doses. Otherwise, side effects may occur and it may become very difficult to safely wean patients off this product. It is also important to increase the cortisol dosage when the body is more stressed. Never stop cortisol suddenly.

• Bio-identical hormone pellet treatment is very useful in helping menopausal women to recover from adrenal fatigue as both estrogen and progesterone help people sleep better and reduce anxiety. Testosterone can improve energy production and mental clarity, making it easier to handle day to day tasks.

Adrenal fatigue is very common. People have mild adrenal fatigue are able to recover from this condition with adequate sleep and lifestyle changes. People with moderate to severe cases can still recover, but it will take more work and time. They need to take the supplements we discussed above for at least six to twelve months and combine them with lifestyle changes.

Points to Remember

1. Adrenal fatigue is very common, especially around mid-life. It is due to long- term physical and/or emotional stress.
2. There are different stages (arousal, adaptation and exhaustion), and different degrees of adrenal fatigue (mild, moderate, and severe).
3. The major symptom of adrenal fatigue is fatigue. Symptoms can range from difficulty getting up in the morning to not being able to function at all. It may also be associated with other diagnoses such as chronic fatigue syndrome, fibromyalgia, hypothyroidism, irritable bowel syndrome, chronic insomnia, diabetes, anxiety, or depression.
4. The diagnosis of adrenal fatigue can be challenging. Saliva testing for cortisol four times a day is the current recommended test. Checking blood cortisol to DHEA ratio is another method.
5. The treatment of adrenal fatigue focuses on stress reduction, improving quality of sleep, a healthy diet to reduce inflammation, and the avoidance of blood sugar fluctuation.
6. Those with moderate to severe adrenal fatigue need supplements to help the adrenal glands produce adrenal hormones. This includes high doses of vitamins such as C, B complex and E, also trace minerals such as magnesium, zinc, and selenium.
7. Herbs and adrenal cell extract helps to support and rebuild the adrenal glands.
8. The adrenal hormone cortisol is available by prescription but has to be used with caution and reserved for patients with severe adrenal fatigue.
9. Consider bio-identical hormone treatment, especially the implanted pellet form, if you are menopausal with adrenal fatigue.

Chapter 7

Hypothyroidism — The Hidden Epidemic

Anna's story —

My name is Anna, age fifty-seven. About ten years ago, I was diagnosed with hypothyroidism (low levels of thyroid hormone) by my family practitioner in North Carolina. She told me I had the thyroid of an eighty-year-old and treated me with thyroid replacement hormone. A few months later, I relocated to Florida. My new doctor thought my thyroid was okay and discontinued it. So, I thought my problem had been corrected. Thereafter, my health gradually began to decline, until a few years later I no longer had energy to do the things I enjoyed in my daily life.

I could not maintain my strenuous workout routine, a daily activity alternating between resistance training and cardiovascular exercise. I caught every flu and cold bug circulating in my professional and social environment, and I stayed sick much longer than normal. I was losing so much hair, the vacuum cleaner clogged every time I swept the carpet. I was more sensitive to cold. I gained weight, even though I ate a very healthy, carb-conscious diet. All of these symptoms were compounded by the fact that I also entered menopause, which I thought was the culprit for my decline. I certainly had the typical hot flashes and night sweats that accompany its onset. My quality of life plummeted. Some mornings, as I drove out of my driveway headed toward a very busy day at the office, I cried because I was already so totally exhausted. I simply could not imagine how I would make it through the day.

I went to great lengths to research my health problem, spending thousands of dollars and expending a few years trying to get to the bottom of my difficulties, with no clear-cut results. Then, I heard about bio-identical replacement hormones that were in the form of pellets implanted in the rear hip area. The physician who managed this treatment was one of only three doctors in Florida to do so, but fortunately just minutes from my home. When he reviewed my lab work, he confirmed "at long last" my low thyroid hormone levels were contributing to my health problems.

As an adjunct to pellet implantation, he prescribed 30 mg daily of Armour thyroid and subsequently raised it to 60 mg. Since then, I have lost thirty pounds, my energy levels have returned to normal, I no longer shed hair at prodigious rates, and I am able to maintain the active lifestyle I prefer. The combination of hormone pellets and thyroid medication has given me back the quality of life that I so deeply missed during the five years that it took for me to find the reason for my physical decline. No more eighty-year-old thyroids in my fifty-seven-year-old body, thank goodness!

Hypothyroidism

Our hormones work together. The thyroid, ovaries (women), testicles (men), and adrenal glands are particularly related to each other and have overlapping functions. All three hormone glands contribute to energy production, mood, mental clarity, libido, sleep, and weight. By the time men and women reach midlife, it is quite typical for the adrenal and thyroid glands to become overworked due to the stresses of daily living, environmental toxins, and the aging process. Many people, especially women, are diagnosed with thyroid problems. But, like Anna, even more are just approaching the threshold of diagnosis and spend years suffering without knowing they have mild hypothyroidism, or subclinical hypothyroidism.

Hypothyroidism affects our bodies from head to toe, impacting all of the body's major systems and contributing to chronic diseases. Amazingly, millions of people with hypothyroidism do not show any signs or symptoms and go undiagnosed for years with this problem. According to the American Association of Clinical Endocrinologists (AACE), subclinical (borderline) hypothyroidism — or early stages of decline of the thyroid — is a common disorder, affecting anywhere from 1 to 10 percent of the adult population, with greater impact on women. Furthermore, the AACE says that as much as 20 percent of the population over the age of sixty is affected by this silent condition. That means one in five in this age group is afflicted.

In order to better understand this often undetected health problem, let us first look at how the thyroid works.

Functions of Thyroid Hormones

The thyroid gland is shaped like the letter "H" or, better yet, like a butterfly. The central connection of the left and right lobes, or wings, of the gland and sits just below the Adam's apple (voice box), right up against the windpipe. The two wings fit snugly onto the sides of the windpipe.

Thyroid hormones increase the metabolic activities of almost all the cells in the body in a very complicated way. This gland's elaborate revving up of our cells keeps our bodies humming.

Thyroid hormones increase the number of mitochondria within our cells. Think of the mitochondria as tiny power plants that generate energy for cellular activities. If the mitochondria are deficient due to low levels of thyroid hormone, cells do not receive the energy they need to properly function. That is why fatigue is a major symptom of low thyroid levels.

When children are lacking in thyroid hormones, their development is adversely impacted. These hormones are absolutely essential to prevent the stunting of growth in children, including mental retardation.

Thyroid hormones also affect our digestive system by stimulating carbohydrate and fat metabolism. They increase the absorption of glucose (sugar) from the intestines and break down the glucose to generate energy. In addition, they decrease the body's tendency to store fat by increasing the oxidation (breakdown) of fatty acids. Low thyroid hormones contribute to elevated levels of cholesterol and triglycerides, which can clog the arteries and lead to atherosclerosis. When the thyroid gland is working well, it tends to increase cholesterol excretion in the bile. It is important to know that with thyroid replacement medications, cholesterol and triglyceride levels diminish.

Thyroid hormones impact the gastrointestinal system in other ways, as well. They stimulate peristaltic motion (intestinal muscle rhythm to move fecal matter through the bowels) and the secretion of digestive enzymes. Low thyroid levels lead to constipation and indigestion.

The body's basic metabolic rate is governed by the thyroid. One of the most reliable indicators of hypothyroidism is a low body temperature. A healthy thyroid increases blood vessel blood flow, cardiac output, and increases the number of heart beats per minute. An extremely low thyroid function leads to heart failure.

Brain function also relies on a healthy thyroid system. Low thyroid leads to depression, slow thinking, and excessive sleepiness.

Our muscular systems rely on healthy levels of thyroid hormones for increased strength and tone. Low thyroid levels cause muscle weakness.

The normal functioning of the reproductive systems are also impacted by the thyroid gland. Lack of thyroid hormones in women leads to low libido (sex drive), infertility, and irregular menstrual periods. Men will have decreased libido, as well.

Causes of Hypothyroidism

There are several factors that cause the thyroid glands to malfunction, or to slow down their release of thyroid hormones.

First, there are genetic causes. Much like diabetes, thyroid problems tend to run in families, especially in women. If our mothers, grandmothers, or sisters have thyroid problems, it is highly likely we will have those problems too.

A second cause of hypothyroidism occurs when our immune systems malfunction. The immune system normally produces antibodies to attack foreign invaders, usually proteins from bacteria or viruses. But sometimes our immune systems become confused and produce antibodies that attack our own bodies' cells, targeting different organs.

For example, Hashimoto's thyroiditis — also known as chronic lymphocytic thyroiditis — results from these attacks of a person's own immune system on the thyroid gland. This leads to the underperformance of the thyroid gland known as hypothyroidism. Conversely, Graves' disease, which also results from an abnormal immune system attacking the thyroid stimulating function, causes hyperthyroidism or the overproduction of thyroid hormones. I recommend that you have your physician examine and/or test you for food allergies, especially gluten and environmental toxins. It is my belief that the autoimmune process is related to these.

In the case of Hashimoto's thyroiditis, the thyroid hormone initially leaks out of the thyroid gland and elevates thyroid levels. But as the thyroid gland is destroyed over time, hypothyroidism sets in. In most of these individuals, the thyroid hormone levels have not been high enough to cause symptoms of hyperthyroidism. Instead, they are diagnosed with hypothyroidism when the thyroid gland reaches a stage of destruction where it is no longer generating enough hormones.

Iodine is the nutrient our body uses to make thyroid hormones. Iodine deficiency occurs only in areas where the water supply lacks iodine, and should not be common now due to the wide availability of sea salt and seafood. However, it is estimated 25 percent of women have low iodine levels in their bodies. There are several different causes, such as restricted salt intake in the case of hypertension, drinking distilled water, or exposure to chlorine, bromide, or fluoride, which can compete with iodine and reduce iodine absorption into the thyroid gland. A deficiency in iodine often leads to goiter.

Another significant factor contributing to hypothyroidism comes from the adverse effects of environmental toxins. There is not sufficient data to know for certain the long term effects of common chemicals in our environment that infiltrate our bodies. But there are many toxins that have been implicated. These toxins have infiltrated our food and water supplies; namely, pesticides, plastics, and PCBs (polychlorinated biphenyls) that are used as coolants and flame retardants in many household products.[57,58,59] An accumulation of these active synthetic chemicals in our bodies leads to the disruption of the physiologic function of our own hormones, including the thyroid hormones.

Other environmental sources of toxins come from chlorine or bromine added to the water in our hot tubs and swimming pools, and from chlorine, bromine or fluorides added to our drinking water. With the abundance of fluorides in our tap water and in the toothpaste we use every day for the prevention of cavities, our bodies are more likely to accumulate higher levels of these chemicals, which contribute to the slowing of thyroid activity.

A rare condition that can cause hypothyroidism is when the pituitary gland, the master hormone gland located at the base of the brain, underperforms. The pituitary gland secretes thyroid stimulating hormone (TSH) to stimulate thyroid gland to make thyroid hormone. Low levels of TSH cause the thyroid gland to slow down, which then reduces hormone levels.

Symptoms of Hyperthyroidism

- Weight gain or difficulty losing weight
- Sleepiness
- Sluggish thinking, poor memory and concentration
- Depression and anxiety
- Constipation
- Cold intolerance, cold hands and feet
- Loss of sex drive (libido)
- Headache/ migraine
- Aches and pains in muscles or joints
- Irregular periods
- Hoarseness
- Low body temperature
- High cholesterol levels
- Dry skin and brittle nails

Signs of Hypothyroidism

- Hair loss or thinning of eyebrows
- Delayed relaxation of deep tendon reflexes
- Infertility
- Myxedema (a skin and tissue disorder that leads to puffiness around the eyes, swollen lips, thickening of the nose, non-pitting edema, and yellow skin)

Diseases Frequently Associated with Hypothyroidism

The thyroid gland is central to the healthy functioning of the entire body. When it malfunctions as with hypothyroidism, it can contribute to the onset of other debilitating diseases, such as:

- Diabetes mellitus/insulin resistance/obesity
- Chronic fatigue syndrome
- Fibromyalgia
- Allergy or multiple chemical sensitivities
- Autoimmune diseases such as celiac disease, lupus or rheumatoid arthritis
- Depression
- High cholesterol, hypertension and heart diseases
- Chronic joint pain and arthritis
- Menopause
- Infertility

Diagnosis of Hypothyroidism

During my training as an internal medicine specialist, I was taught that there were several tests for hypothyroidism but we only needed to check the levels of thyroid stimulating hormone (TSH). TSH is secreted by the pituitary gland to regulate thyroid function, and if this regulating hormone is found to be in the normal range, there is no thyroid problem.

This sounds simple enough, but in reality many patients have signs and symptoms of hypothyroidism even when lab results show normal ranges of TSH. This is what occurred with Anna, whose new doctor viewed her as a hypochondriac when she insisted her thyroid was the cause of her health problems.

Years after my residency training, I learned that TSH is not an accurate test for hypothyroidism. Our thyroid gland secretes T4 (thyroxin, which is tyrosine with four molecules of iodine). T4 is not an active hormone, so after it enters into the cell one iodine is removed forming T3 (triiodothyronine), which is the active form of the hormone. However, there are many factors affecting the conversion of T4 to T3 and sometimes T4 becomes reverse T3 (the wrong iodine is broken off) instead of normal T3. This explains why the TSH test may be normal as the T4 seems adequate, yet the patient has signs and symptoms of hypothyroidism due to the underlying fact that T3 levels are still low.

Research shows that emotional stress or physical illness blocks the conversion of T4 to T3. Patients with adrenal fatigue usually show normal T4 but reduced T3. Other conditions that can reduce T4 conversion to T3 are unstable blood sugar and insulin levels, autoimmune thyroiditis, mineral deficiencies, and certain drugs.

In my practice I use several tests to check thyroid function. These tests include TSH, free T3 (triiodothyronine), and free T4 (thyroxine). Thyroid antibodies, such as anti TPO, are checked for the possibility of auto immune thyroiditis. From my clinical experience, patients with high anti TPO titer usually have food allergies. I have many patients who, after avoiding the foods they are allergic to, find that the anti TPO titer lowers and their thyroid function improves!

Another very important but simple diagnostic tool involves charting the basal body temperature when a patient has signs and symptoms of hypothyroidism. The patient's body temperature is taken immediately upon awakening before engaging in any physical activity. If it is consistently lower than 98° F, chances are the thyroid function is low.

In addition, if I detect lumpiness or thyroid gland enlargement (goiter) just below the patient's Adam's apple, I obtain an ultrasound scan to check for thyroid nodules or other abnormalities.

Treating Hypothyroidism

1. Medication —

The first successful treatment of hypothyroidism was recorded in 1891 in England with the use of desiccated porcine (pig) thyroid gland extract. This was the most effective form of treatment until the 1960s, when pharmaceutical companies began mass production of medications to simulate T4. This treatment has since dominated the medical treatment of hypothyroidism and is prescribed under such brand names as Synthroid, Levoxyl, and Unithyroid.

These medications, however, are not cure-alls for hypothyroidism. The problem is that T4 needs to be converted in the body to T3 to perform thyroid hormonal functions. A pharmaceutical firm subsequently developed Cytomel, a patented T3, to help patients who do not respond well to the T4 medications. But Cytomel is short acting and needs to be taken twice a day.

Interestingly, the original medication, desiccated porcine thyroid, which is now prescribed as Armour thyroid, seems to be quite effective. A study published in 2001 followed eighty-nine patients who were taking T4 medications and then switched to desiccated thyroid.[60] They were followed for two years and their symptoms of hypothyroidism were then compared to their symptoms before the switch. Fatigue dropped from 90 percent to 26 percent; constipation, from 40 percent to 14 percent; depression, from 61 percent to 23 percent; and cold intolerance dropped from 86 percent to 24 percent.

It is fascinating to note that the symptoms of hypothyroidism did not greatly improve with previously administered T4 medications. With desiccated thyroid, however, there was remarkable improvement in all symptom categories. The reason is probably the existence of T3 and other thyroid hormones, T1 and T2, which may have their own therapeutic functions too. But remember, everyone is different. Environmental toxins can block the cascade of endocrine and immune actions, making some individuals very sensitive to even small doses of thyroid medication. Other hormones such as sex hormones and adrenal hormones also affect thyroid hormones; people with adrenal fatigue can react adversely to thyroid hormones unless they also receive adrenal hormones at the same time. Or, like in Anna's case, they are treated with female bio-identical hormones and thyroid hormone simultaneously. Anna, who opted to take this route, experienced a phenomenal rebound.

Sometimes we may have to try different thyroid medications until the desired result is achieved. It is also important to take thyroid medication on an empty stomach because foods, especially those high in calcium, reduce the absorption of thyroid hormone.

2.   Nutrition —

A patient with hypothyroidism may benefit from nutritional supplements, such as tyrosine, selenium, iodine, zinc, and magnesium, but thyroid hormone medication is usually the first choice of treatment since thyroid hormones affect digestion. A person suffering from hypothyroidism does not digest or absorb nutrients well.

In addition to thyroid medications, however, a balanced and healthy diet is always recommended. Some foods and substances should be avoided entirely, as they can directly interfere with thyroid function, such as impeding the conversion of T4 to T3. These are caffeine, alcohol, tobacco and sugar.

Specific foods, such as seaweed (kelp) and seafood are important for thyroid hormone production. They contain the trace minerals such as selenium, zinc, iodine and proteins that are needed for the manufacture of thyroid hormones. Replacing table salt with sea salt is another simple way to get iodine.

I recommend the nutritional supplements in the following daily dosages: tyrosine (100mg), zinc (20 mg); selenium (200 mcg); and iodine (150 mg). Herbs, such as ashagandha may improve the conversion of T4 to T3.

3.   Detoxification

As mentioned before, thyroid hormones are interrupted by many environmental toxins, such as pesticides, plastics, heavy metals, and water with fluoride and chlorine. Toxin avoidance is the first step, followed by detoxification as discussed in Chapter 11. It is important to improve constipation by using more fiber, magnesium, and the proper dose of thyroid hormones, as fecal excretion is one of the major routes of detoxification and many patients with low thyroid function have constipation problems. If you have Hashimoto's due to auto antibody attack on thyroid glands, avoiding foods that you are allergic to is very important as this will reduce the antibody titer and thus reduce the attack on thyroid glands.

4.   Stress Reduction

When stressed, our adrenal glands secret higher levels of cortisol. These higher levels inhibit the conversion of T4 to T3, leading to a reduction in the levels of the active form of the thyroid hormone, T3.

5.   Hormone Balance

All hormones work together. Thyroid hormones are particularly affected by adrenal and sex hormones. Optimize those hormones and you will feel wonderful again.

Self-assessment for Hypothyroidism

Here is a simple test to help you determine if your thyroid gland is functioning optimally.

1.   Do you often experience fatigue? Do you wake up feeling tired even with a good night sleep?

2.   Do you have cold hands and feet? Do you often need to wear socks to bed?

3.   Do you have trouble losing weight, even with little food and lots of exercise?

4.   Are you mentally sluggish, forgetful, or mentally foggy?

5.   Do any of your family members have thyroid problems?

6.   Do you suffer from dry skin, brittle nails, or hair loss?

7.   Do you have irregular periods or difficulty getting pregnant?

8.   Do you have multiple allergies or chemical sensitivities?

9.   Do you have chronic constipation and/or indigestion?

10.   Do you have bouts of depression or anxiety?

If you answered "yes" to more than four questions, it increases the likelihood that you may have borderline or undetected hypothyroidism.

Points to Remember

1. A normal thyroid function test result does not exclude the diagnosis of hypothyroidism.

2. Signs, symptoms, and family history of thyroid problems support a diagnosis.

3. Menopause, adrenal fatigue, and hypothyroidism often occur simultaneously.

4. Many factors can affect the conversion of T4 to T3, the active thyroid hormone.

5. Avoid environmental toxins as much as possible in order to prevent a deleterious effect on the thyroid gland.

6. Avoid fluoridated tap water and toothpaste with fluorides.

7. Avoid exposure to chlorinated water in swimming pools or hot tubs.

8. T4 treatment alone is often ineffective. Many people need a mix of T3 and T4.

Chapter 8

Regenerative Medicine

Human Growth Hormone and Stem Cell Treatment

In recent years there has been a growing amount of media attention and consumer interest in the use of human growth hormone (HGH). Advertisers have been quick to tout the benefits of these substances, claiming a wide variety of benefits which encompass everything from enhanced sports performance to slowing down the aging process. Stem cell treatment sparked so much interest both for medical communities and general public as the fountain of youth and the future of medicine. In this chapter we are going to take an in-depth look at the scientific facts behind HGH and stem cell treatment.

Human Growth Hormone

HGH is a protein structure made up of 191 amino acids secreted by the pituitary gland in the brain. The function of HGH is to promote growth by helping the transportation of amino acids into cells, and the synthesis of amino acids into new cellular structures, especially bones and muscles, as well as internal organs. It is essential in childhood and our young adult years for the purpose of growing bigger and taller. HGH secretion reaches its peak by a person's late teens and declines gradually after that. By the age of sixty or seventy, we only have 15 to 20 percent of the hormone levels we had in our peak years.

Since all adults stop growing at some point, it makes sense to ask: Why would we still need HGH in our older years if we are not growing anymore? The answer can be found in HGH's primary function, the synthesis of amino acids. HGH is still needed to help our bodies use the amino acids we ingest to repair cellular damage and generate new cells.

There are quite a few benefits claimed by those who use HGH supplements. Some of these benefits include younger looking skin, stronger bones and immune system, improved muscle mass and cardiac output, increased energy, enhanced sexual performance, sharpened memory, and balanced mood. If some of these benefits sound strangely familiar to you, it is because we have been talking about them in conjunction with pellet therapy all along. As a matter of fact, similar effects can be achieved by implanted bio-identical estrogen and testosterone pellets, which are also hormones that promote growth.

Recent news headlines reported that high profile athletes in Florida were using HGH illegally in an attempt to improve their sports performance. However, the truth of the matter is that in adults with normal levels of growth hormone, raising levels too high will cause problems like carpel tunnel syndrome, diabetes, or even acromegaly, a medical term for enlargement of bones in the jaw, hands, and feet.

But what about claims that HGH slows down the aging process in men and women? Is growth hormone really the fountain of youth everyone has been searching for? In my opinion, before the age of sixty, hormone replacement with testosterone and/or estradiol pellets will accomplish all this, as they have been proven to improve energy, memory, sexual performance, muscle strength and exercise endurance. After age sixty, there may be a role for HGH replacement, but only after all other hormones, such as thyroid, adrenal and sex hormones, are balanced and in good range. For those individuals who do choose HGH therapy, it is important to always use a physiological dose, monitor hormone levels regularly as high dose HGH causes side effects under the care and treatment of a physician.

One drawback to HGH replacement is its high cost and inconvenient application. Because HGH has 191 amino acids, making it a fairly large molecule, it is not able to enter our body through the skin or digestive tract. The only way to receive HGH is through daily subcutaneous injections, just like insulin given to patients with diabetes. The cost is also very high, about $500 to $1,000 a month depending on the dosage used.

What most people do not realize is that there are natural ways to increase the amount of HGH our body produces. Proper nutrition and daily exercise are the two primary vehicles by which our body can naturally increase HGH production and the amount it releases. We know that nutrients and amino acids such as arginine, ornithine, tyrosine, and methionine contribute to HGH production and release. Strenuous aerobic exercise thirty minutes daily also stimulates the release of growth hormone. By exercising daily and putting wholesome, nutritious foods in your diet you are well on your way to assisting your body in optimal HGH production. For patients who have yet to do this, I recommend starting an exercise program, preferably with a strong aerobic component, and taking amino acid supplements in the morning before exercise.

Stem Cell Treatment

What is stem cell? —

The first stem cell is the embryo being formed after fertilization. It has the capacity to transform into different tissues, such as nerve, muscle, skin, bone, blood, and organs such as brain, lung, pancreas, lung, and heart. After we are born, we have stems cells stored in different part of our body and can be used to generate new cells where they reside when needed. As we age, the stem cell storage declines.

There are different types of stem cells:

1. Embryonic stem cells: this is the most potent stem cell that can transform to any types of cell as needed. Embryonic stem cell research was banned in the USA for eight years and was lifted in 2008.

2. Adult stem cells: this can be derived from umbilical cord, abdominal fatty tissue and bone marrow. Those cells are more differentiated and more limited as to what cells and organs they can become.

Stem cells share two properties:

1. Self-renewal: the ability to go through numerous cycles of cell division while maintaining the undifferentiated states.
2. Potency: the ability to differentiate into different cell types.

Types of stem cell treatment:

1. Autologus stem cells. These stem cells are harvested from our own body, such as bone marrow or abdominal fatty tissue. The bone marrow aspiration can be painful and has more potential side effects. Abdominal fat is easier and safer to harvest through liposuction and will generate more stem cells.
2. Allogenic stem cells. These stem cells are harvested from another person. This can be from new born baby's umbilical cord or by using embryonic stem cells.

Safety and effectiveness of stem cell treatment:

Safety of stem cell treatment is related to the type of cell and the manipulation involved. Manipulation includes expansion (cultured and expanded to more cells), storage (freezing), and purification. The less manipulation of stem cell results in safer stem cell treatment. If you use the autologus stem cell, which is your own, it's safer than the allogenic stem cell. Adult stem cells are safer than embryonic stem cell because it is more technically challenging to control the behavior of embryonic stem cell.

The effectiveness of the treatment is related to the potency and quality of the stem cells. Unfortunately, potency is generally the reverse of safety. For instance, the embryonic stem cell is the most potent but the least safe one to use. The quality of stem cell depends on the laboratory that can produce cells with high potency and safety consistency. In Asia there are now clinics that met the USA's FDA standards for stem cell quality. Earlier in this book I told you that I have tried stem cell therapy in my desire for increased energy and improved hormone levels. I found that some Asian clinics have medical specialists schooled and trained in America — many from our highly ranked medical schools. I found the experience to be first rate and the treatment to be highly beneficial.

The potential of adipose stem cells in regenerative medicine:

As we discussed above, using autologus stem cells harvested from abdominal fat is the safest stem cell treatment at this time. Since adult stem cells do have limitation as to what they can differentiate into, let's take a look at what adipose stem cells are capable of.

Adipose stem cell is a mesenchymal stem cell which can develop into bone, muscle, tendons, ligament, fat, and internal organs such as lung, liver, pancreas, heart, and hormone gland. It also has an immunomodulatory function. This function helps the body fight autoimmune diseases such as rheumatoid arthritis, Crohn's disease and multiple sclerosis.

The safety and efficiency of adult stem cell for tissue regeneration is currently under assessment in clinical trials. There are studies around the world using adult stem cells to treat conditions such as type 1 diabetes, liver cirrhosis, hepatitis, cardiovascular diseases, autoimmune diseases, and neurodegenerative diseases.

The objective of stem cell research is to dramatically change and improve medical treatments for many serious diseases and ailments. The goal is to achieve a higher quality of life for all. Think about it; what if you were facing a future of doubt, pain, and medical problems due to the need for a new kidney; however, you could regenerate your own. What if you needed insulin due to type 1 diabetes yet you could now produce your own and eliminate external insulin shots? What if you could prolong your youthfulness by rejuvenating your own hormone glands? All of these and more may be possible from stem cell research. This is truly an exciting time we live in!

I strongly believe stem cell research for medical use will be available soon for many more of us that can benefit from this treatment. However, I want the reader to remember that a strong and consistent foundation for personal health must first be followed. Let us not forget that a seed will not grow in poor soil. We must improve our diets, exercise, limit stress, and follow a plan of regular medical examinations. We must also teach our children these foundations so they may pass it on to their children.

Part III: The Body, Mind, and Spirit Connection

Chapter 9

Nutrition — You Are What You Eat

There are all kinds of diets: the Zone diet, Pritikin diet, South Beach diet, Mediterranean diet, Okinawa diet, low-fat diet, low carb diet, and vegan diet. The list goes on and on. For a long time, it has been considered sinful to eat fat. Now everyone is shying away from carbohydrates and sugar. So, what is left to eat?

Consider the nutrients derived from food. They are carbohydrates, proteins, fats, vitamins, minerals, enzymes, and fibers. All carbohydrates turn into sugar (glucose) as the source of immediate energy for the body. All proteins turn into amino acids, which are the building blocks of cellular structures, hormones and neurotransmitters. Fats turn into fatty acids, which are also building blocks for cellular structures and hormones in the body. Vitamins and minerals are involved in all of the body's chemical reactions, including the detoxification systems. The body secretes enzymes to digest food, and, fortunately many fruits and vegetables are also loaded with enzymes to help digestion. Fibers help with the elimination of solid wastes. Thus, all of the nutrient groups have their functions, and including each group in our diet is important for our optimal health.

While the basic nutrient groups have remained the same over the millennia, the way humans eat has changed significantly over the past fifty years. As a result of this, problems occur because we have altered our diet from the way that was designed for us genetically over millions of years of evolution. Unlike our primitive ancestors, we eat food that has been processed, refined, bleached, radiated and loaded with food colors and preservatives. We eat food that is even grown differently, due to commercial farming practices that rely on artificial fertilizers, toxic pesticides, and in some cases, genetic modification. This food, unfortunately, generally has a much lower nutritional value than the more natural foods that our ancestors ate. Our food not only gives us poorer nutrients, but is also laced with substances that are toxic to our health. Worse yet, we overeat and our bodies turn this excess of calories into fat.

Let us look more closely at how the nutrient groups in food work in the body.

Breakdown on Nutrients

Carbohydrates:

Carbohydrates are made of sugar molecules chained together. There are two types of carbohydrates: simple and complex. Complex carbohydrates are made of three or more sugar molecules chained together, while simple carbohydrates are just one, or two connected sugar molecules.

Complex carbohydrates are found in whole grains, vegetables, and legumes. Examples of simple carbohydrates are fruits, cookies, cakes, and candy. All carbohydrates are broken down in the digestive tract and then absorbed as sugar. Simple carbohydrates, with shorter chains of connection, break down more quickly and are absorbed right away.

Processed carbohydrates come from foods that are refined, such as grains or starchy vegetables. For instance, brown rice is converted to white rice when the outer shell is stripped away. The outer shell contains fiber (the complex carbohydrate), which must be broken down by digestive enzymes before the inside of the rice kernel can be digested. Eating white rice causes the blood sugar to rise much faster than eating brown rice. However, in the end, both the brown rice and white rice produce the same amount of sugar.

Another example of refinement is processing the potato into potato chips. In the body, they both convert to sugar fairly fast, but potato chips have other ingredients, such as salt, hydrogenated oil, and preservatives that are not good for the body. Also in the process of refinement, the vitamins and enzymes in the potato are destroyed.

The glycemic index has been developed as a tool to measure how quickly the body converts carbohydrates into sugar. The amount of food ingested also matters. The index, times the amount, comes to the total glycemic load. If you eat a small piece of candy, which has high glycemic index, compared to a bowl of rice, which has lower glycemic index but a higher total amount of carbohydrate, the total glycemic load will be higher in the bowl of rice.

The glycemic index, however, is not the only measure of how fast sugar is absorbed. When we combine foods in a meal, such as fiber, protein or fat, the absorption of sugar will be slowed down due to competition for absorption sites in the small intestine. That is why a balanced meal is important.

The key is to eat mostly complex carbohydrates, not the refined foods that alter complex carbohydrates to less healthy and more quickly absorbed simple carbohydrates. Another key is not to overeat. Too much intake of carbohydrates will only be turned into fat and stored in the body, which leads to weight gain and insulin resistance.

Examples of sources of good carbohydrates, both complex and simple, are:

- Starchy vegetables: carrots, beets, potatoes, yams, corn, and peas.

- Leafy vegetables: spinach, lettuce, cabbage, chard, and kale.

- Grains: barley, brown rice, millet, oats, quinoa, rye, and whole grain wheat.

- Fruit: apples, bananas, berries, oranges, lemons, watermelons, and papaya.

Fats:

Many people think eating fat will make you fat. This is a myth. The fact is the body needs good fats, which become fatty acids that are used to make cellular structures and hormones. The undesirable fat that we gain is usually due to eating excessive simple carbohydrates.

Fatty Acids:

- Fatty acids are the building blocks of fat. All fatty acids are made of long chains of carbon molecules that have to bind with hydrogen molecules. There are three types of fat: saturated, monounsaturated and polyunsaturated.

- Saturated fat: All the carbon atoms are saturated with hydrogen atoms. Sources of saturated fats are butter, cheese, eggs, coconut oil, and fatty tissue from animal meat.

- Monounsaturated fat: One site is missing a hydrogen atom. Sources of monounsaturated fats are almond oil, avocado oil, olive oil, grape seed oil, and canola oil.

- Polyunsaturated fat: More than one site is missing hydrogen atoms. Sources of polyunsaturated fats are flaxseed oil, sesame seed oil, evening primrose oil, wheat germ oil, corn oil, and fish oil.

- Essential Fatty Acids

Among the polyunsaturated fats, there are three essential fatty acids: omega-3 fatty acids, omega-6 fatty acids, and gamma-linolenic acid. The term "essential" means that the body cannot make these fatty acids and we need to get them through our diet. These polyunsaturated fats are essential for our hormone production, particularly the prostaglandins, a group of hormones found in virtually all of the tissues and organs of the body. Prostaglandins act as inflammatory mediators, constrict smooth muscles, and sensitize spinal neurons to pain. Lack of essential fatty acids will lead to more inflammation and aging, in part, because the production of good prostaglandins is slowed. Omega-3 is also the building block for cell membrane structures and nervous system formation. Sources of essential fatty acids:

- Omega-3 fatty acids: flaxseed oil, walnut oil, and fish oil from salmon, sardines, tuna, and mackerel.

- Omega-6 fatty acids: canola oil, flaxseed oil, grape seed oil, corn oil, sunflower seed oil, chicken, eggs, and turkey.

- Gamma-linolenic acid: borage oil, evening primrose oil, and blue green algae.

Bad Fat:

There are good fats and bad fats. All naturally occurring fats are good fats. Bad fats are damaged fats, usually as a result of refinement processes used to manufacture them. They include:

1. Hydrogenated Oil

    a. This is manufactured by adding an extra hydrogen atom to vegetable oil, which results in an oil that is a liquid in its natural form but becomes solid at room temperature. Margarines and shortenings are examples of hydrogenated oil.

2. Trans-fats

    a. Polyunsaturated fats are good for the body, but when processed with high heat they become trans-fats and bad for the body. When extracted with heat, corn oil, for instance, becomes a trans-fat. If it is cold pressed, which means that it is manufactured without the use of heat, then it is good for the body. So, always buy vegetable oils that are cold pressed.

    b. French fries and fried foods are loaded with trans-fats due to cooking the food with high heat. Most of the polyunsaturated oils cannot withstand high heat, so do not cook with flaxseed oil or sesame seed oil. Instead, use them in salad dressing. The best cooking oil is saturated fat, such as butter or coconut oil, because it is stable when heated. Grape seed oil can also tolerate higher levels of heat in cooking.

3. Oxidized, Rancid Oil

    a. When oil is exposed to air, oxygen binds with the carbon atoms and the oil becomes oxidized. This changes the color of oil as well as its taste and smell. All oil should be refrigerated after opening. Do not use oil that has been opened and sitting in the cabinet for over three months.

    b. When bad fats get into the body, they replace the natural fat in the cell membrane and make it more rigid. The cell membrane is the gateway to all nutrients and hormones. If the cell membrane malfunctions, such as when it becomes more rigid, the nutrients and hormones the cell needs cannot enter. Bad fat also becomes debris that clogs our cells and blood vessels, which leads to atherosclerosis and premature aging.

We usually get enough omega-6 fatty acids from foods like chicken, turkey, or eggs. Conversely, we usually do not get enough omega-3 fatty acids from our diet, so supplementation is important.

Protein:

All protein turns into amino acids and becomes the building blocks for muscles, bones, organs and tissues. The amino acids are also precursors to neurotransmitters. As such, protein is essential for life. There are twenty amino acids in protein. About ten are essential amino acids. This means that the body cannot make them, so they have to come from our diet. Good protein usually comes with good fat.

Sources of good protein are:

- Eggs: You can eat one to two eggs daily. Do not worry about the impact on cholesterol levels. Ninety percent of cholesterol is made by the liver, not derived from dietary sources of cholesterol.

- Meat and poultry: Always buy organic or hormone free meat and poultry. Do not buy processed meat, such as sausages or ham that come loaded with nitrates and preservatives.

- Fish and shellfish: Buy fresh fish instead of canned or smoked varieties. It is preferable to consume wild fish or smaller fish in order to avoid mercury. Farmed salmon is often fed dyes to color its meat.

- Cheese: Most cheese is treated with heat, which can damage its fat, so eat it with moderation. Avoid yellow cheese, as it is colored with dye. Buy organic cheese. People who are allergic to milk cannot eat cheese.

- Nuts and seeds: They are excellent sources of good protein and good fat. Nut butters are processed, so be careful about preservatives. Nuts are best eaten raw after soaking for eight hours, which will activate their enzymes for easy digestion. Examples of nuts and seeds are almonds, walnuts, cashews, chestnuts, macadamia nuts, peanuts, hazelnuts, pistachio nuts, pecans, pine nuts, sunflower seeds, sesame seeds, and pumpkin seeds. You can grind nuts and seeds, then add olive oil and sea salt to use as a salad dressing or a vegetable dip.

Vitamins:

- Vitamin A
  o Vitamin A is important for healthy vision and healthy skin. This vitamin is found in both animals and plants.
  o Animal sources of vitamin A are beef, liver, and butter.
  o Plant sources are yellow colored fruits and vegetables, such as yams, pumpkins, carrots, and apricots.
- Vitamin B
  o Vitamin B is composed of eight water-soluble vitamins, including B1 (thiamine), B2 (riboflavin), B3 (niacin), B5 (pantothenic acid), B6 (pyridoxine), B7 (biotin, also called vitamin H), B9 (folic acid) and B12 (cyanocobalamin). The B vitamins are also found in animals and plants. These vitamins are essential for cell functions, especially in the central nervous system. A deficiency of the B vitamins can lead to such diseases as anemia, nerve cell damage, fatigue, PMS (premenstrual syndrome), hormonal imbalance, and malabsorption.
  o Animal sources of vitamin B are chicken, fish, pork, beef, eggs, and milk.

- o Plant sources are nuts, seeds, lentils, whole grains, potatoes, leafy green vegetables, corn, mushrooms, broccoli, and beans.

- Vitamin C

  - o Vitamin C is important for wound healing and immunity. It helps with the formation of collagen and maintaining youthful skin. Collagen is the main component of fascia, cartilage, ligaments, tendons, bone and teeth. Vitamin C is also a strong antioxidant that neutralizes the free radicals that lead to inflammation. Thus, it slows down the aging process and also plays an important role in the body's detoxification process.

  - o Vitamin C deficiency leads to increased bruising, poor wound healing, and scurvy. Scurvy leads to spongy gums and bleeding from all mucous membranes, as well as the formation of liver spots on the skin. As the disease progresses, individuals lose their teeth and have open, pus-filled wounds.

  - o Sources of vitamin C come from plants only. Humans cannot make vitamin C, and depend on foods such as citrus fruits, cantaloupes, tomatoes, cabbage, and broccoli as a source of this vitamin.

- Vitamin E

  - o Vitamin E is an important antioxidant that helps stabilize cell membranes. It protects against lipid peroxidation, which is the breaking down of cell membranes. Vitamins C and E work together to reduce inflammation and to prevent atherosclerosis (hardening of the arteries). There are eight forms of vitamin E. The most common is alpha tocopherol, but delta and gamma tocopherol also have synergistic effects.

  - o Deficiency of vitamin E leads to cellular oxidation and to formation of plaque in the arteries. Vitamin E is important for cardiovascular and brain health.

o   Animal sources of vitamin E are egg yolks and various fats.

o   Plant sources are leafy green vegetables, vegetable oils, whole grains, and legumes.

- Vitamin D

o   Vitamin D plays an important role in the absorption of minerals, such as calcium, magnesium and phosphorus. Vitamin D deficiency leads to osteoporosis. Recent studies suggest that vitamin D may protect against autoimmune diseases, such as multiple sclerosis, and different forms of cancer, including breast, colon and prostate.

o   Low vitamin D is also associated with mood issues such as depression.

o   Vitamin D is produced by exposure of our skin cells to the sun. Food sources are cod liver oil, liver, and egg yolks. Milk and many cereals are fortified with vitamin D.

Minerals:

- Calcium

o   Calcium is important for healthy bones and teeth, but it's most important role is in the cell membrane for activating enzymes, neurotransmitters, and hormones.

o   Calcium is also involved with nerve conduction, muscle contraction, blood pressure regulation, and many other metabolic functions. One type of blood pressure medication is called a calcium channel blocker, which blocks the influx of calcium into cells and reduces blood pressure.

o   Because calcium is so important for many life preserving activities; when it is needed, the body will pull the calcium stored in bones for use in the circulatory system. Thus, insufficient calcium leads to osteoporosis.

- o Animal sources of calcium are fish or sardines with bones, chicken, milk, cheese, yogurt, and egg yolks.
- o Plant sources are tofu, beans, broccoli, green vegetables, nuts, and seeds.

- Magnesium
  - o Magnesium is also a very important mineral because it involves important metabolic functions, especially energy production in the mitochondria (energy units inside cells). Magnesium relaxes muscles, reduces blood pressure, prevents constipation, and improves mood and sleep. Magnesium deficiency leads to an irregular heartbeat, muscle spasms or pain, irritability, and nervousness.
  - o Magnesium is primarily derived from plants such as beans, broccoli, and avocados, as well as fruits such as lemons, apples, figs, and grapefruits.
  - o In my practice I use chelated magnesium (400-800 mg daily) to treat many conditions such as palpitations, high blood pressure, constipation, muscle cramps, insomnia, and anxiety.

- Chromium
  - o Chromium is involved in glucose metabolism and has been shown to improve insulin sensitivity (increases the body's response to insulin so less is required). This makes it a very important supplement for people who have diabetes or sugar craving.
  - o Animal sources are meats, eggs, and cheese.
  - o Plant sources are nuts, mushrooms, beets, and legumes.

- Selenium
  - o Selenium works with vitamin E and helps in stabilizing the cell membrane. It is also an antioxidant involved in liver detoxification. Studies

show selenium helps prevent cancer, diabetes, and heart diseases. It also boosts one's immunity.

o   Selenium deficiency is often due to heavy metals that can inactivate this mineral. Heavy metals that interfere with its function include cadmium as a result of smoking or exposure to batteries, mercury from eating certain fish or as a result of dental amalgam fillings, and/or lead due to exposure to industrial and automobile pollution. Animal sources of selenium are tuna, salmon, meats, and other seafood. Plant sources are fresh garlic, wheat germ, whole grains, and mushrooms.

- Zinc

o   Zinc is another essential antioxidant mineral that is involved in many cellular functions and enzyme pathways. Studies show that zinc helps to protect the eyes from blindness due to macular degeneration, improves arthritic conditions, and enhances immune function. Animal sources are chicken, pork, turkey, beef, liver, eggs, seafood, and milk. Plant sources are wheat germ and pumpkin seeds.

- Iodine

o   Iodine is very important in the production and regulation of thyroid hormones. Low levels of iodine lead to hypothyroidism and goiter (enlarged thyroid gland). Iodine is also involved in many enzyme systems involving energy production, nerve function, breast health, hair, and skin growth.

o   The best food source is seaweed, especially kelp, sea salt, and iodized salt.

- Potassium

o   Potassium plays a major role in maintaining tiny electrical currents in the cells, especially heart and muscle contractions, and nerve transmission. Low potassium levels lead to an irregular heartbeat, muscle cramps, weakness, and even mental confusion.

o   The best food sources for potassium are fruits like bananas and oranges. Other plant sources are apricots, lettuce, broccoli, potatoes, nuts, seeds, wheat germ, and other fresh fruits.

o   Animal sources are liver and fish.

- Iron

o   Iron is essential for the formation of hemoglobin, which carries oxygen from the lungs via red blood cells to the body. Iron is also found in myoglobulin, a molecule in the muscles that transports oxygen to muscle tissue. A lack of iron leads to anemia, which is more common in women before menopause.

o   Animal sources of iron are liver, meats, and shellfish.

o   Plant sources are leafy green vegetables, whole grains, fruits, and nuts.

- Fiber

o   Fiber is the structural material of plants that performs a function similar to the skeletal structure of animals. It is important for the GI (gastrointestinal) tract, as it is the food source of friendly bacteria in the large intestine. There are two types of fiber: water soluble and water insoluble.

o   Fiber is found in all plant sources such as fruits and vegetables, whole grains, nuts, seeds and legumes.

- Water-soluble fiber

o   Water-soluble fiber plays several important roles:

▪   It slows down the entry of carbohydrates into the blood stream, thus it reduces blood sugar and insulin secretion. That is why eating water-soluble fiber from vegetables is very important for individuals with diabetes or insulin resistance.

- Helps detoxification by binding heavy metals and other toxins.

- Helps to lower cholesterol by binding the cholesterol in the bile and food. Sources of water soluble fibers are vegetables, fruits such as apple, and carrots. The mucilage of legumes and seeds also contain water-soluble fibers.

  o Water insoluble fiber has very little effect on sugar absorption or insulin secretion. It does increase the bulk of stool, which helps with elimination, detoxification, and preventing constipation.

Enzymes:

The body secretes enzymes to digest food. Many fruits and vegetables contain enzymes that help with digestion. Cooking food at a temperature over 118° F will destroy the enzymes provided in food. In fact, cooking food at a temperature above 160° F will destroy all vitamins in the food. This is why we should attempt to eat the majority of our fruits and vegetables raw.

Water:

Up to 70 percent of the body is made of water, which really is our number one nutrient. There are two types of water in the body: intracellular water and extracellular water.

- Intercellular Water

  o Intracellular water is water within the cell and is needed for all cellular functions. More water is maintained in the cells (over 60 percent of the total) the younger we are. As we age, we maintain less intracellular water. That is why children's skin looks like freshly picked grapes, while seniors look like raisins. Less intracellular water leads to reduced cellular function and lowered metabolism. The cell membrane determines whether or not water can get into the cell. A soft membrane is more water permeable, while a rigid one is not.

o To improve intracellular water, we need to improve cell membrane permeability by eating foods with more omega-3 essential fatty acids, as they are building blocks of cell membranes. Another factor is toxins in the body, because more toxins in the tissue draw water out of the cell. Removing toxins by detoxifying the body will help the permeability of the cell membrane.

- Extracellular Water

  o Extracellular water is the water that circulates in the bloodstream and between cells. Too much extracellular water leads to water retention and edema. Not enough water in the circulatory system causes dehydration, which has serious consequences such as fatigue, weakness, light-headedness, and fainting.

Water quality is also a problem. It is not a good idea to drink tap water, as chlorine and fluoride are added to the water supply. Other chemicals, such as fertilizers, pesticides, as well as organic chemicals such as PCBs and benzene can leak into the water supply from the environment. The quality of drinking water can be controlled by installing a home water filtration system, such as reverse osmosis or multi-stage carbon filter.

Whatever your health goal is, you can customize your diet to fit your needs. The principle of a healthy diet is one that gives us adequate nutrition and also reduces inflammation.

Anti-inflammation Diet

There are six key concepts to reduce inflammation:

1. Avoid sugar and refined carbohydrates. High glycemic index carbohydrates increase blood sugar and thus trigger insulin secretion. High insulin triggers inflammation reactions.

2. Reduce toxins in the food and water.

   o Avoid processed foods, which have artificial food colors, sweeteners, preservatives, and MSG.

    o   Eat organic foods to avoid pesticides, herbicides, and xenohormones.

    o   Drink filtered water and use glass or stainless steel container.

3.   Increase omega-3 fatty acids from salmon, avocados, nuts, or seeds to reduce inflammation. Avoid trans-fats, hydrogenated oil and rancid oil from foods such as hamburger and french fries which cause inflammation of blood vessels and rigid cell membrane.

4.   Increase antioxidants from fruits and vegetables of all colors. Antioxidants neutralize free radicals and reduce inflammation.

5.   Increase fiber and water to assist the body's detoxification processes.

6.   Use herbs such as ginger, garlic, rosemary, and turmeric, which have an anti- inflammation effect.

Weight Loss Diet

1.   Reduce your total calorie intake. Check your metabolic rate. Most people will be able to lose weight with a diet of 1,000 to 1,400 calories a day.

2.   Our body prefers to use sugar as our energy source. If you keep on eating carbohydrates, you are not going to burn fat. It is a good idea to eat mostly protein initially to switch our body's energy utilization system.

3.   Drink lots of filtered water (50 percent of your body weight in ounces). This helps with detoxification and reduces hunger feelings.

4.   Avoid high glycemic index carbohydrates, especially from refined white flour products such as pastas, cakes, cookies, pretzels, donuts, white bread, white rice, pizza, noodles, etc. Avoid foods loaded with sugar, including candies, baked goods, fruit juices, soft drinks, ice cream, etc. These foods stimulate insulin secretion and the more you eat the hungrier you get. This is a big "NO NO" if you want to lose weight and improve metabolic syndrome.

5.   Avoid bad fats from processed foods (potato chips, popcorn, etc.), fried foods (french fries, fried chicken, etc.), processed meats (bacon, sausages, hot dogs, ham, smoked or cured meats, etc.), rancid oil, trans-fats, and saturated fats.

6.   Eat the fresh organic vegetables listed below as much as you like. Eat them mostly raw. Vegetables provide abundant enzymes, antioxidants, minerals and fiber. Cooking destroys enzymes and vitamins.

   a.   Green leafy and cruciferous vegetables are: alfalfa sprouts, broccoli, cabbage, cauliflower, chard, collard greens, kale, lettuce, and spinach.

   b.   Other vegetables are asparagus, bell peppers, celery, cucumbers, green beans, mushrooms, onions, peas, radishes, string beans, sprouts, summer and winter squash, tomatoes, zucchini, and sea vegetables (kelp).

7.   Eat good protein and good fat, such as organic nuts, seeds, avocados, chicken, turkey, and wild salmon. Remember the serving size, not more than three ounces, and the methods of cooking include baking, broiling, and grilling.

8.   You can have whole grains (oatmeal, brown rice, millet, etc.), fruits (apple, berries, oranges, grapes, pineapples, etc.), and legumes (garbanzo beans, kidney beans, black beans, lentils, etc.), but eat only one group at each meal and be careful about your portions. These foods are healthy, but they still contain quite a bit of carbohydrates.

9.   Condiments: Cinnamon improves insulin sensitivity, so use it generously. Turmeric, ginger and garlic have anti-inflammation effects, so use them frequently too.

10.   Eat small frequent meals. Avoid eating a large dinner or eating late at night.

Many of my patients tell me that they eat a healthy diet, but still cannot lose weight. Once the hormones are balanced, they lose weight naturally. Another reason people can't lose weight is due to toxin overload and food allergies. Once this is addressed, weight comes off easily too.

Healthy Aging Diet

1. Reduce inflammation, as discussed above.

2. Do not overeat. A famous study done in 1935 showed the life span of laboratory rats could be extended by 50 percent with serious calorie restriction. While in humans this can be unrealistic, the goal of avoiding overeating is achievable.

3. Choose your fat wisely. Essential fatty acids, especially omega-3 fatty acids, are used to make hormones and cellular structures. Increasing good fats, such as avocado, supplements of fish oil, flaxseed oil, along with nuts and seeds, helps to increase hormone production, improves immunity, and reduces inflammation.

4. Increase growth hormone production by increasing the intake of amino acids, such as protein shakes, especially before exercise.

5. Optimize digestion and absorption by eating raw fruits and vegetables that come with enzymes. Eat fermented food such as yogurt or sauerkraut for the healthy bacteria that protect the intestinal tract. Have vinegar with salad to increase the stomach acidity. Remember that old and wise saying: eat slowly, enjoy your food and thoroughly chew all your food.

Alkaline Diet

The measurement of acidity or alkalinity of a media is called pH. The scale is from 0 to 14 and 7.0 being neutral pH under 7.0 is acidic while over 7.0 is alkaline. Our bodies keep a very narrow pH range, from 7.35 to 7.45. A slightly changed pH environment will affect the chemical reactions in our body so the body will try everything to maintain a stable pH environment. I remember when I was working in the ICU; many times I had to draw arterial blood to measure the pH. Since those patients were critically ill, they lost the ability to regulate the pH and we had to give IV sodium bicarbonate to correct metabolic acidosis, which is very common in critically ill patients.

Foods are digested and broken down into either an acidic or an alkaline end product. Foods that produce an alkaline end product are called alkaline forming foods while foods that produce an acidic end product are called acid forming foods. It is important to note that certain foods, such as lemons, can be highly acidic and can form alkaline end products in our body.

Acid forming foods include meats, cheese, sugars, eggs, coffee, and white flour. Artificial sweetener such as NutraSweet and Equal (aspartame) are extremely acid forming. Diet soda is particularly acid forming and should be avoided.

Alkaline forming foods are fruits, vegetables and herbal teas. Alkaline water has been popular in recent years but can it really make a difference? Our stomach is the only part of our body that is very acidic. Once the alkaline water enters the stomach, it will neutralize the stomach acidity but the stomach will produce more acid into the lumen, thus pull out more acidity from our body. So it is good to drink alkaline water but don't drink it with meals, as we need acidity in the stomach to digest the food, drink it in between meals.

Our body will pull the minerals out of our bones to neutralize the acidity so the pH can be maintained. This is why drinking milk does not help with bone density. We need to eat more alkaline forming foods than acid forming food, which means more fruits and vegetables and less meats, dairy and processed foods.

Points to Remember

1.   Eat balanced meals, as all nutrients have important functions.
2.   Eat smaller meals, snack in between meals if you are hungry.
3.   Never overeat, but do eat when you are hungry.
4.   Reduce inflammation by avoiding high intake of sugars and fatty foods.
5.   Eat foods in their natural forms and try to avoid processed or refined foods. Eliminate artificial food colors, sweeteners, and preservatives.
6.   Eat fresh organic fruits and vegetables of all colors.

7.   Cooking destroys enzymes and vitamins; eat raw vegetables and sprouted foods for their increased nutritional value and supply of enzymes.

8.   Eat fresh organic nuts and seeds as sources of proteins and beneficial fats.

9.   Eat unprocessed organic meat, eggs, chicken, butter, and wild salmon.

10. Eat fermented foods, such as yogurt, soy yogurt, sauerkraut, and miso soup to promote friendly bacteria in the intestinal tract.

11. Avoid trans-fats, hydrogenated oils, and rancid oils. Avoid cooking with vegetable oils and use organic butter or coconut oil instead. Avoid all deep fried foods.

12. Buy cold-pressed vegetable oils.

13. Avoid high-glycemic index carbohydrates, especially processed foods made of white flours and sugar.

14. Drink plenty of filtered water. Aim to drink 50 percent of your body weight in ounces each day.

15. Fibers help the body to detoxify, as well as reduce cholesterol, slow down the absorption of sugar, and lower the release of insulin. All fruits, vegetables, and whole grains provide fiber.

16. Add herbs such as garlic, ginger, cinnamon, and turmeric for seasoning because of their high nutritional value and anti-inflammation effect.

17. I highly suggest eating more alkaline forming foods such as fruits and vegetables. I also suggest avoiding acid forming foods such as meats, dairy and processed foods. I further suggest avoiding all sodas and especially diet sodas. Try to replace sodas with herbal teas.

Chapter 10

Intestinal Health — Our First Line of Defense

The GI Tract

Good nutrition depends not just on what we eat, but also on how healthy the GI (gastrointestinal) tract is. The GI tract has a surface area 200 times greater than our skin and is exposed to the external environment via the foods we eat. Your GI tract is actually a highly evolved ecosystem. Inside a healthy GI tract are over 1000 trillion microflora that live, thrive and create a healthy GI tract. These microflora assist in vitamin production and nutrients creation which become the energy source for the gut lining. The microflora form a slick layer on the surface of your intestines so large food molecules and/or toxins cannot enter our body. When this ecosystem is disrupted, or the intestine tract becomes inflamed, harmful substances can enter our bodies and create negative immune responses that, in turn, could create Crohn's disease or food allergies.

Components of the GI Tract

The GI tract is a major system of the body and consists of:

- Mouth and Teeth
    - o The functions of the mouth and teeth are receiving food, chewing to break the food down into smaller particles and mixing these particles with saliva, which secretes enzymes to split complex

carbohydrates (starches). It is important to chew food thoroughly and to keep your teeth and gums healthy. A poor state of oral health where loose and lost teeth are common will adversely affect your ability to chew thoroughly. Infection in the gums can cause low-grade inflammation and even heart valve infection.

- Esophagus
  o The main function of the esophagus is to swallow so that chewed food will move from the mouth down to the stomach. The epiglottis is an elastic cartilage tissue that sits over the vocal cords. It closes during swallowing to prevent food from going down the windpipe and causing choking. This is a very serious risk for the elderly because choking can cause aspiration pneumonia, which results from accidentally inhaling food or liquids. Avoid talking or laughing when your mouth is full.

- Stomach
  o The stomach further mixes chewed and salivated food into chime, and digests protein by secreting HCl (hydrochloric acid) as well as the enzyme pepsin. The stomach only digests proteins, not carbohydrates or fats.

- Pancreas
  o The pancreas manufactures and releases digestive enzymes. Pancreatic enzymes are released via the pancreatic duct into the duodenum (first part of the small intestine beyond the stomach) for the digestion of foods. The enzymes trypsin and chymotrypsin digest protein into amino acids; amylase digests starch into sugar; and lipase digests fat into fatty acids. Insulin is also secreted by the pancreas to handle the sugar load in food and to help transport the sugar from the bloodstream into the cells.

- Liver
  - o The liver is the chemical factory of the body. After all the foods we eat are digested and absorbed, the nutrients go directly to the liver, where sugar is converted into glycogen to be stored as a future energy source. The liver also converts the glycogen back into sugar for use when the body requires it. The liver stores vitamins such as vitamin A, D, E, K, and B12. It manufactures bile to store in the gallbladder. The liver is also the body's major detoxification center. It converts fat soluble toxins into water soluble forms, so the toxins can be carried through the bloodstream to the kidneys for excretion in the urine or through the bile duct to the intestines to be eliminated as stools (feces).
- Gallbladder
  - o This is the storage place for bile, which emulsifies fat. People who have gall stones or have their gallbladders taken out may have problems digesting fat and may develop bloating and diarrhea.
- Small Intestine
  - o The small intestine has three sections: the duodenum, jejunum, and ileum. The final breakdown of fats, proteins, and carbohydrates takes place in the duodenum. Ninety percent of the absorption of nutrients occurs in the jejunum and ileum. Problems in this area will lead to malabsorption and malnutrition.
- Large Intestine
  - o The horseshoe shaped large intestine consists of the ascending colon, transverse colon, and the descending colon. The major function of the large intestine is absorbing water, short chain fatty acids, and vitamins produced by beneficial bacteria in the colon. The large intestine also eliminates feces.

Beneficial Bacteria

At birth, the GI tract is sterile. Shortly thereafter, bacteria start to colonize the large intestine. These friendly bacteria are symbiotic with the body. Their total number exceeds that of our own cells. They feed on the fiber we eat and produce fatty acids and vitamins, particularly the B complex vitamins, for use by our bodies. They form a slimy layer on the intestine wall, where they help to prevent the overgrowth of yeast, viruses, and toxic bacteria.

The protection provided by healthy bacteria is very important. As we age, beneficial bacteria decrease in number. They are also destroyed by frequently taking antibiotics, having frequent intestinal infections or food poisoning. At such times, it is important to reintroduce friendly bacteria by eating fermented foods such as sauerkraut, yogurt, or soy yogurt. Taking probiotics (healthy bacteria such as acidophilus) also helps.

We need to eat twenty-five to thirty-five grams of fiber each day to feed friendly bacteria. Since the body produces a lesser amount of enzymes and absorbs fewer nutrients with aging, it is also a good idea to take digestive enzymes in pill form to aid with the digestion of food.

GERD

GERD means gastroesophageal reflux disease. The lower esophageal sphincter is located at the junction of esophagus and stomach. It prevents the stomach content from moving back to the esophagus when the sphincter is closed completely. However, many factors can cause the sphincter not closing tightly, so the acidic stomach content goes back to the esophagus, so called reflux, thus leads to heartburn, indigestion, and belching.

Common causes of reduced esophageal sphincter tone include:

1. Foods with high fat, sugar, caffeine or food allergies.
2. Overeating, obesity, smoking or alcohol use
3. Delayed gastric emptying due to inadequate acid or pepsin secretion and improper digestion.
4. Lying down or bending after eating.

Over-the-counter antacids and medicines, such as Zantac or Prilosec (proton pump inhibitor), are most commonly used to treat bloating, gas, dyspepsia (heartburn), and acid reflux. However, they only work by reducing the stomach acidity so that stomach content flowing back no longer cause irritation. This does not address the issues that causes of reduced esophageal tone. Long term use of antacids interfere with the digestion of important nutrients, such as amino acids, which is the building block of neurotransmitters and cellular structures. Gastric acidity is required to kill the harmful bacteria. Low gastric acidity can lead to infections. The real treatment for GERD has to address the cause of it. Here are some simple life style changes you can use:

1.   Eat small meals. Avoid eating large meals near bed time.
2.   Avoid lying down immediately after eating.
3.   Avoid, or limit foods with high fat, simple sugar, and caffeine containing beverages.
4.   Begin a weight loss program.
5.   Avoid acidic foods such as orange juice, citrus fruits, and alcohol
6.   Stop or limit smoking
7.   Elevate the head of your bed to prevent reflux

By adapting these life style changes many of my patients have eliminated their use of antacids and prescription medicines. Some patients have even eliminated their chronic heartburn by using herbs, vitamins and minerals to restore a healthy gastric lining. My preference is aloe vera, slippery elm, zinc, glutamine and the combination referred to as DGL (deglycer rhized licorice root). Each of these can be taken in simple pill form and are readily available at most health food stores. For my patients with acid reflux I recommend a gluten and dairy free diet.

Leaky Gut Syndrome and Food

Allergies:

This is a group of disorders not usually emphasized in medical textbooks. Most doctors are not very aware of this disease category. Yet, patients with this problem suffer tremendously. They go from doctor to doctor without getting the right diagnosis or treatment. The more problems they have, the more medications that are prescribed for them, and pretty soon they become walking pharmacies. Unfortunately, this predicament only tends to make the sick become sicker.

How do people get this type of disease? It starts either from a dysfunctional gut or from excessive exposure to toxins, and in many instances the combination of both. We absorb nutrients through two pathways: diffusion and active transport. Diffusion is a simple process. Substances of different concentration equilibrate and reach the same concentration. Electrolytes, such as sodium, potassium, magnesium, bicarbonate, and chloride get into the body in this way. But most nutrients such as amino acids, fatty acids, glucose, minerals, and vitamins enter the body through active transport, which means the body produces carrier molecules that actively carry the nutrients into the intestinal cells. The linings are very tight between the cells so that large molecules or unwanted substances cannot make their way into the body. Think of this as a secured gate of a house, which only opens for guests but not for uninvited people. When uninvited people enter the house, the alarm will be activated and a fight will begin to take place. When unwanted foreign molecules or large food particles get into the body, the body produces antibodies to fight those molecules. This process causes inflammation.

Leaky gut is a disease syndrome caused by an impaired intestinal defense system that allows toxins, large undigested food molecules, unwanted chemicals and microbes to get into the body. This then triggers all kinds of diseases and symptoms, ranging from allergies, acne, asthma, autism, eczema, irritable bowel syndrome, ulcerative colitis, autoimmune diseases, arthritis, headaches, fibromyalgia, mood swings, foggy mind, memory loss, multiple chemical sensitivities, and premature aging.

There are several ways that the body's intestinal defense system is impaired or destroyed, which can then cause a leaky gut:

1. Antibiotics

    a. The first antibiotic, penicillin, was discovered in 1928 by Scottish scientist Sir Arthur Fleming and later developed for use as a medicine by Australian Nobel Laureate Howard Walter Florey. Penicillin saved the lives of many people who would have otherwise died from infectious diseases. After that, numerous antibiotics were manufactured. Now they are given liberally whenever we have a cold, flu, bronchitis, sinusitis or urinary tract infection. These antibiotics kill both good and bad bacteria, so that long term or frequent use of antibiotics destroys the protective healthy intestinal bacteria and opens the door to the overgrowth of resistant bacteria, parasites, viruses, and fungi such as candida. These unhealthy microbes often form chemicals that are poisons in the body, such as ammonia, hydrogen sulfide, indoles, and phenols that not only damage the intestinal mucosa lining but also enter into the bloodstream, causing a large variety of diseases and symptoms.

b.   Candida is a fungus found in our environment and in the body. It is normally kept under control by friendly bacteria, the immune system and the intestinal pH. When candida anchor and colonize the intestinal mucosa, they secrete toxins that enter into the bloodstream directly. These toxins contribute to inflammation, bloating, fatigue, headache, mental fog, and other symptoms. They also damage the intestinal cell lining so that large undigested food molecules can enter the bloodstream, which triggers the formation of antibodies. While these antibodies are working to fight the food molecules, they can also damage our own tissues, and cause autoimmune diseases.

2. Pain Medications

a.   NSAIDs (non-steroidal anti-inflammatory drugs) such as aspirin, Advil®, Motrin®, Aleve® and ibuprofen are the most commonly sold over-the-counter (OTC) medications.

b.   Prescription medications such as Naprosen, indomethacin, Voltaren, Toradol, and Celebrex® are also in this group. The latter are more potent than the OTC pain medications.

c.   NSAIDs work by blocking prostaglandins, which are a group of hormones involved in the body's process of healing and repair. Certain prostaglandins can also increase inflammation and pain. Accordingly, there are good and bad prostaglandins. NSAIDs indiscriminately block all of them. They reduce pain by blocking the prostaglandins that increase pain and inflammation, but they also block the prostaglandins that improve healing and repair, including the intestinal linings, where the cells turn over every three to five days. Thus, one of the well-known side effects of NSAIDs is GI irritation, ulcers, and bleeding. Long-term use of NSAIDs will interfere with the healing and repair of the intestine lining and may cause a host of other problems.

3.   Poor Eating Habits and Lifestyle

    a.   Our diet has a tremendous impact on our GI system:

        i.   A low-fiber diet makes us prone to constipation. As a result, toxins reside longer in the intestines and irritate the intestinal mucosa.

        ii.   Processed foods loaded with sugars, hydrogenated oil, trans- fatty acids, food colors, artificial sweeteners and preservatives promote inflammation of the intestinal lining.

        iii.   Alcohol and the use of multiple drugs affect the liver's detoxification function and contribute to the accumulation of more toxins in the body, which damages cells in the intestinal lining.

        iv.   A stressful and sedentary lifestyle reduces the immune defense system and flow of blood to the intestines. In the long run, every cell in the body is affected and does not function optimally. This includes the intestinal lining cells, especially since they are regenerated every three to five days.

4.   Environmental Toxins

    a.   The body can only handle so many toxins. If we are continually bombarded with environmental chemicals and heavy metals our bodies will eventually be overwhelmed with toxins. These toxins interfere with cellular functions, including those of the intestinal lining. When the intestinal defense system is lowered, more toxins enter the body. It becomes a vicious cycle.

5. Other Medications and Treatments

    a. Steroids such as prednisone or cortisone are used frequently to treat allergies and autoimmune diseases. Long-term use of these medications suppresses the immune system and increases fungus growth in the GI tract and other parts of the body.

    b. Radiation to the abdominal area as a cancer treatment can damage the intestinal mucosa and cause leaky gut. Most chemotherapy drugs damage the body's cells and the GI tract. This leads to such side effects as nausea, vomiting, and malabsorption.

Diagnosis of Leaky Gut Syndrome

Determining the presence of leaky-gut syndrome involves a combination of the following tests.

1. Intestine Permeability Testing

    a. Both mannitol and lactulose are complex sugar molecules that the body cannot utilize or metabolize. Once ingested and absorbed, they are excreted in the urine unchanged. Mannitol is much smaller than lactulose. A healthy intestine absorbs mannitol easily, but not so with lactulose. Patients with leaky gut absorb a much higher ratio of lactulose compared to healthy people. The test is done by drinking a mannitol and lactulose solution. The urine is collected for six hours and then sent to the laboratory. A high ratio of lactulose/mannitol indicates the permeability of the intestine is too high, which is consistent with a leaky gut.

2. Comprehensive Digestive Stool Analysis (CDSA)

    a. This test measures the bacterial balance of the intestinal tract and digestive functions. It checks the types of bacteria that are present and measures the levels of beneficial and harmful bacteria. It also checks for the presence of candida and what therapeutic agent is most effective. This test also checks the butyric acid and short chain fatty acids that are produced by friendly bacteria in the intestines. A low level of short chain fatty acids means an insufficient amount of probiotics (friendly bacteria). Checking for parasites can also be done with the CDSA, but the result can be unreliable if just done on one random sample. Multiple testing will increase the reliability of the accuracy of the results.

3. Food Allergy Testing

    a. Allergists usually do skin testing or blood testing for IgE antibody-mediated allergies, such as hay fever or asthma. But most food allergies are not IgE antibody mediated. Checking IgG antibodies is more reliable for food allergies. Other antibodies, such as the antiglidin antibody for wheat allergy and the antibody for candida can be checked with food allergy panels, which can include up to 150 different foods.

Treatment of Leaky Gut Syndrome

The diagnostic tests can be expensive and may not be covered by insurance companies, so a course of treatment can be tried first to see if there is improvement clinically.

1. Assist Digestion of Food

    a. Chew your food well and take digestive enzymes with each meal. This is the easiest and least expensive method of treatment. Digestion starts in the mouth. As we chew, digestive enzymes from saliva are mixing with the food. If you chew the food into smaller particles, it makes the work of the stomach and small intestines much more efficient. Taking digestive enzymes with each meal further aids with digestion and reduces large food molecules as they move into the intestinal walls.

2. Avoid Common Food Allergens

a. Avoid common food allergens. Eighty percent of food allergies are due to diary, wheat, processed foods, and citrus fruits. You can simply do an elimination diet, by eating only rice, all fruits except citrus fruits, all vegetables except nightshade vegetables (tomatoes, eggplant, potatoes, and red/green/yellow/ chili peppers), fresh herbs (garlic, ginger, oregano, parsley, dill, rosemary, thyme, turmeric), fish, chicken and olive oil. Drink only filtered or mineral water or herbal tea. Eliminate alcohol, soft drinks, coffee, decaffeinated coffee, chocolate, red meats, soy and soy products (tofu, soy milk, soybeans), milk and milk products (ice cream, cheese, cottage cheese, butter, yogurt, cream, and baked food with milk), wheat and wheat products (bread, pasta, cereal, and crackers), all processed foods, artificial sweeteners and condiments. Once you feel better, start introducing one type of food at a time, such as red meat, nuts, seeds or soy products. Introduce one new food and eat it two to three times a day. If you are feeling fine after a few days, introduce another type. If your old symptoms return, you are probably allergic to this type of food. Once you find the food you are allergic to, avoid it for at least six months and reintroduce afterward. If you get sick again, you may have to permanently eliminate this type of food, which will most likely be milk or wheat products. Finding the foods you are allergic to in this way is very cost effective. It does take time, patience and persistence to do it correctly.

3. Treat Dysbiosis

a. Dysbiosis is due to the imbalance of intestinal bacteria flora. There are three types of bacteria: the helpful, the neutral, and the harmful. When there are more harmful bacteria than helpful bacteria, your health is jeopardized. Treatment depends on the type of pathogens you have. Your physician should be able to prescribe the appropriate medication after stool testing. Natural treatments that are effective to eliminate pathogens are garlic, grapefruit seed extract, and oil of oregano in capsules. Candida also responds to natural treatment. A prescription antifungal medication sometimes kills the candida too quickly and large amounts of endotoxins are released into the bloodstream. This will worsen a patient's symptoms. It is a good idea to use a small dosage to begin and gradually increase the dosage as needed.

4. Reintroduce Friendly Bacteria

   a. Dr. Eli Metchnikoff was a scientist who was awarded the Nobel Prize in 1908 for discovering the friendly bacteria called lactobacilli, which can displace many disease producing bacteria and reduce the toxins they generate. Lactobacilli (found mostly in the small intestines) and bifidobacteria (found mostly in the large intestines) are the two most well studied friendly bacteria. Humans and friendly bacteria are symbiotic; we supply them with a warm environment and lots of foods (fibers), and in return they produce vitamins that include B1, B2, B3, B5, B6, B12, and folic acids. They also produce lactic acid, which facilitates the absorption of minerals such as calcium, iron, and magnesium. The lactic acid and hydrogen peroxide that these friendly bacteria produce inhibit other harmful microbes. Take probiotics supplements that contain lactobacilli and bifidobacteria, one to two capsules two to three times a day. Most of them need to be refrigerated to keep the bacteria alive. Eating yogurt or soy yogurt helps, but you need a much higher count of friendly bacteria if you have dysbiosis.

b.   Japanese researchers have studied fructooligosaccharides (FOS) and found those sugar molecules can rapidly increase the growth of lactobacilli and bifidobacteria. Many foods have FOS, especially bananas, barley, garlic, onions, asparagus, tomatoes, and artichokes. Taking probiotics together with foods high in FOS will double the effect.

5.   Reduce Toxins

a.   Reduce exposure to toxic substances and use antioxidants to help the body detoxify. Please see Chapter 11 for greater detail.

6.   Healthy Diet

a.   See Chapter 9 for more information on nutrition.

Candida

Candida is a form of yeast that is harmful to our body. Normally the GI tract has a healthy balance of bacteria and yeast. Under certain conditions, such as overuse of antibiotics or long term consumption of foods high in sugar, Candida albicans increase rapidly in its fungal form and grow over the beneficial bacteria. This causes GI inflammation, food allergies, and leaky gut and they can secrete toxins directly into our body. The symptoms can be non-specific. In the intestine tract, most common symptoms are gas, bloating, and constipation. Due to the toxins secreted into our body, we can have fatigue, mental fog, weight gain, sugar craving, headache, skin rash, allergies, or just not feeling well.

The treatment starts with diet which is the most important treatment. Without proper diet, candida will come back quickly even if it's killed with medication. Another very important treatment is healthy bacteria and yeast to suppress the growth of candida. I also have my patients use prescription anti-fungal medication or nutritional product that has an anti-fungal effect.

Diet guidelines:

1.   Candida thrives on sugar, so eliminate sugar and simple carbohydrates such as honey, corn syrup, sucrose, maltose,

lactose, maple syrup, white flour, potato and corn chips. Avoid processed foods, such as cakes, cookies, candies, bread, and pasta. Fruits and starch vegetables such as potato or yam can be consumed in small quantities.

2.   Avoid fermented foods such as cheese, wine, beer, and alcoholic drinks.

3.   Avoid baked foods such as bread and pastry.

4.   Eat fresh food. Do not eat leftover food that has been in the refrigerator more than two days.

Self-assessment for Leaky Gut

Use this questionnaire to gauge your current state of intestinal health. Answer each question based on the following symptoms:

Point scale:
0 = not present
1 = mild and happen sometimes
2 = moderate and happen often
3 = severe and happen all the time

Section A

1.   Do you have constipation and/or diarrhea?

2.   Do you have abdominal pain or bloating?

3.   Do you have indigestion or reflux?

4.   Do you have burping and belching?

5.   Do you have flatulence and passing gas?

6.   Do you have nausea or vomiting?

Total Score for Section A

Section B

1.   Do you have stomach discomfort when consuming certain foods?

2.   Do you have blood or mucous in your stool?

3.   Do you pass foul smelling gas or stool?

4. Do you suffer from chronic constipation?

5. Do you experience frequent diarrhea after traveling to another country?

6. Do you have joint pain or swelling?

7. Do you have low energy or become easily fatigued?

8. Do you have hay fever or sinus congestion?

9. Do you have asthma attacks?

10. Do you have ulcerative colitis, Crohn's disease, or celiac disease?

11. Do you have eczema, skin rash or hives?

12. Do you have fibromyalgia or chronic fatigue syndrome?

13. Do you experience mood swings, irritability, mental fog, or memory loss?

14. Do you use antibiotics frequently for urinary tract infection, sinus and respiratory tract infections?

15. Do you use NSAID medications, such as aspirin, Motrin®, Advil®, or Aleve®?

16. Have you engaged in the prolonged use of steroids such as prednisone?

Total Score for Section B

Interpreting the Results

Section A

If you scored four or more in Section A, you will benefit from an intestinal health and repair program. The symptoms are due to suboptimal digestion and inflammation of the GI tract. Taking digestive enzymes, probiotics, and fiber with a diet that reduces inflammation may help. If not, seek professional help.

Section B

If you scored four or more in Section B, you may have intestinal dysbiosis (toxin producing bacteria or yeast in your intestine), food allergies, or leaky gut. You may start the treatment yourself with the plans discussed above. You may also need to seek professional help.

Summary

Hopefully you now see that achieving and maintaining a nutritious and balanced diet is critical in resisting diseases and for your general health and well-being. However, this is only the first step towards improving your health and quality of life. It is just as important to achieve and maintain a healthy GI tract. If you are experiencing, or beginning to experience, any of the symptoms I have already mentioned then it is very important for you to take the necessary steps to restore your intestinal lining back to health.

The easiest way to restore your intestinal lining is to use the "4 R" program. Remove, Replace, Re-inoculate and Repair. This simple formula will pay off handsomely in healthy dividends. When made part of your new lifestyle you will see how easy it is to maintain and how much better you will feel. The first step is to remove from your diet processed, fried and sugary foods. The next step is to replace the digestive factors with Betaine HCL, pepsin, and digestive enzymes. The third step is to reintroduce healthy bacteria to your intestinal tract. The fourth step is to repair the intestinal lining with herbs and amino acids such as DGL, glutamine, N Acetyl systeine, ginger, and turmeric.

If you need help in starting this program, or perhaps you need support and guidance while doing so, I suggest you see a physician or licensed dietician. Once you begin to experience the elimination of former gastric problems you will be able to make this a regular part of your life and I know you will be happy that you made these changes.

Chapter 11

Our Toxic World — The Silent Killer

Bio-identical hormone pellets have helped people to experience remarkable improvements in their quality of life by revitalizing the body, balancing the emotions, and clearing the mind. Sometimes, however, addressing hormonal issues alone is not enough to bring patients back to a state of optimal health. As a physician who encourages patients to look at and consider the entire picture when it comes to their health, I know that our bodies can be susceptible to both internal factors and the environment around us. Each day I see more and more patients who reflect this sensitivity, a powerful reminder that our environment has become increasingly toxic and poses continued risks to our health. Take Mary, for instance, and the journey towards healing that she undertook when her body began to suffer from the toxic effects of mercury poisoning.

Mary's story—

My name is Mary, and at age fifty, my body suddenly "hit the wall." I had previously been extremely active and had been working hard to build and maintain my health as I approached middle-age. I was dedicated to exercising regularly and eating highly nutritious meals. But then I was stricken with a flu that took weeks instead of days from which to recover. I had a lingering cough that just would not go away. My internal medicine doctor diagnosed asthma and prescribed powerful medications that he said I would need to take the rest of my life. After a few weeks, with the irritating cough still persisting, I saw a pulmonary specialist, who told me that I had an asthmatic bronchitis that accompanied the flu virus and was way overmedicated. Nonetheless, he suggested I continue to take the asthma medicine, just at a lower dosage. I did not want to be on that medication at all. Thoroughly disgusted with what I had experienced with these two doctors, I then sought the help of a doctor of Chinese medicine who was able to gradually wean me off of the asthma medicine. Months later, however, after weekly treatments of acupuncture and cupping, she admitted that she could not understand why that nagging cough would not go away. Every time a cold or flu afflicted someone I knew, I caught it and became terribly sick with a severe respiratory infection followed by the lingering cough. After a year of this suffering, I found a naturopath who diagnosed that my real problem was not in my lungs but, rather, it was due to the many dental amalgams in my teeth. He said that my sudden decline in health, persistent cough and respiratory infections, fatigue (which was not relieved by sleep), depression, and hopelessness was due to mercury toxicity. By now my life had become a matter of doing the bare minimum to get by each day. My naturopath referred me to the team of a biological dentist and physician who specialized in mercury detoxification. Having already spent two years and thousands of dollars trying to find the healing journey that entailed as my dentist said, "The replacement of a lifetime of bad dental work in just a month."

Immediately after one or two of the mercury-laced dental amalgams were removed from my teeth, I would go to the physician for IV chelation. This was necessary because, even though my dentist took extraordinary precautions to protect himself, his assistant, and me from exposure to mercury while removing the amalgams, he said that it was impossible for him to prevent incidental exposures. The IV chelation would help my body recover from this toxic exposure. In fact, while my dentist was working on my fillings, a lady visited his office to ask his advice. Having heard of the dangers of mercury toxicity, she had her amalgams removed all at once by a dentist who did not follow the safety protocols practiced by this dentist and physician. She was extremely sick and she hoped that my dentist would be able to help her. With the damage already done, he told her it was unfortunately too late, she would now have to live with it. In my own case, after the completion of the dental work to replace the silver/mercury amalgams with materials that were biologically friendly to my body, my physician told me it would take a year for me to regain my health.

It was a tough year with several setbacks of painful respiratory infections, but it turned out that my doctor was right. Gradually, my energy returned. I was able to get a good night's sleep and wake up in the morning more refreshed. My immune system began to ward off circulating colds and flu. My life returned to normal. A couple of years later, I encountered a man stricken with mercury poisoning who was confined to a wheelchair. Once a powerful executive, he was unable to talk or walk due to the neurological damage caused by this noxious heavy metal. It was quite scary to think that I could have ended up in that predicament had I not aggressively sought the underlying cause for my lung ailments. I am so grateful that I have had the opportunity to properly and safely eliminate the source of my mercury exposure.

Have you ever wondered why there is such an increased rate of breast cancer and prostate cancer compared to fifty years ago? Or why so many people suffer from allergies? Have you ever thought about why diseases such as chronic fatigue syndrome, fibromyalgia, or multiple chemical sensitivities were not even mentioned in medical literature fifty years ago? Or wondered about why so many children are diagnosed with autism or attention deficit hyperactivity disorder (ADHD) when in the past these were rare diseases? Have you ever wondered why there are so many neurodegenerative diseases such as Parkinson's, Alzheimer's, and multiple sclerosis? The last century has borne witness to rapid changes in our level of technology, industry and manufacturing processes, more so than in any other century before. Our use of land for agriculture and development, combined with our high demand for fossil fuels has led to a number of significant changes in the environment, including deforestation and ozone depletion. This, in turn, has had a profound effect on the air we breathe, water we drink, and land we use to produce our food. All of these changes have a direct impact on our health.

Consider the following questions:

- Did you know that the average human sperm count has dropped by more than half, from 125 million/ml in 1932 to 50 million/ml in 1998?

- Did you know that there has been a 30 to 40 percent increase in undescended testes and deformed penises in boys over the past thirty to forty years?

- Did you know that data from the Environmental Protection Agency (EPA) shows that 1.2 billion pounds of chemicals that are potentially harmful to humans were released into the air and water in 1998 alone, and that about four billion pounds of pesticides are now used annually in the U.S.?

- Did you know that, since World War II, between 75,000 and 80,000 new synthetic chemicals have been released into the environment? Did you know that on average, more than 400 synthetic chemicals can be found in your body at any given time?

Human beings are conducting a massive, dangerous experiment to see what the chemicals we have invented will do to our bodies, our environment, and our planet. It is not just one or two chemicals, but hundreds and thousands of them combined together.

Rachel Carson wrote *Silent Spring* in 1962. Carson warned in her visionary book that, unless we change what we are doing, there will also be a silent summer, fall, and winter. She described how the proliferation and persistence of chemicals were contaminating our environment. Carson also documented how those chemicals accumulated in our bodies. Human beings living in such remote areas as Canada's Baffin Island now contaminated with synthetic chemicals such as PCBs, DDT, and dioxin. Since that time, efforts have been made to clean up the environment, but there has not been enough accomplished to alleviate the damage that has accrued over time, nor is enough being done today to prevent further damage.

Three decades after Carson's warnings about the damages accruing from polluting our environment, Theo Colborn, Dianne Dumanoski, and John Peterson Myers wrote *Our Stolen Future* (1996). This book provides scientific research about a wide range of man-play critical roles in our health, and their disruption can lead to low sperm count, infertility, neurological disorders, and hormone-triggered cancers such as breast and prostate cancer.

Faced with this array of evidence documenting the decline of our environment, we need to ask the important questions: Are we threatening our fertility and survival? If so, what should we be doing about it?

Types of Toxins

With the arrival of the Industrial Age, humankind has managed to compound all manner of chemicals, while helpful to the manufacturing of myriad products, also taint the environment and hence our bodies. These include pesticides, industrial compounds, fertilizers, and heavy metals, among others. Let us take a closer look at some of the major toxins in our environment.

Pesticides —

There are three major types of pesticides that have been commonly used over the last century. Many are still in use today.

1. Organochlorides
   a. This is a group of chemicals and pesticides known as chlorinated phenols. The most well-known one is

DDT (dichlorodiphenyltrichloroethane), which was first synthesized in 1874. However, its use as a pesticide did not begin until the 1940s, when it was sprayed to control mosquitoes and protect crops. Chlordane was used in pest control for millions of homes from the 1940s to the late 1980s. Heptachlor replaced chlordane, until it was banned in 1978. Even though these pesticides have been banned, they can persist in our environment for decades. Meanwhile, other pesticides in this group are still being used, such as 2, 4-D and 2, 4, 5-Trichlorophenoxyacetic acid. These numerically named organochlorides are commonly used in agriculture and on lawns.

b. PCP (pentachlorophenol) is used as an outdoor wood preservative for the treatment of utility poles and railroad ties.

c. PCBs and PBBs (polychlorinated biphenols and polybrominated biphenols) were widely used in electrical equipment and transformers in the past and are still used in construction.

d. Chloroform (trichloromethane), discovered in 1831, was originally used as an anesthetic drug, but was banned from use in consumer products in 1976. Yet chlorine in the water combined with organic material such as dead leaves produces chloroform. It is found in water treatment facilities and in tap water in many cities.

e. Carbon tetrachloride can be found in cleaning products, degreasing agents, dry cleaning solutions, and paints. In the 1940s, it was used in refrigerants and fire extinguishers, but such use has since declined. Its use in consumer products was banned in 1970.

This group of chemicals can cause DNA changes and cancers. These chemicals also damage the liver, kidneys, immune system, and central nervous systems.[61]

Even though it has been banned since 1972, DDT can still be found in human breast milk, blood, urine, and sperm. It is also found in many forms of wildlife in many different parts of the planet. In birds, it caused such thin and brittle eggshells that it seriously threatened the survival of several species, including the peregrine falcon.

2.   Organophosphates

    a.   The common group of pesticides, marketed as Dursban, diazinon, parathion, and malathion was designed as a nerve gas to damage the nervous system and kill insects. It can also damage the central nervous system of humans and affect the behavior of both humans and animals, causing symptoms such as blurred vision, confusion, in-coordination, and even death.[61,62] The use of organophosphates has also been linked to brain cancer, leukemia, and non-Hodgkin's lymphoma. Dursban has been used widely over the past twenty years for termite control. It was only partially banned in 2001. This group of pesticides has been spayed liberally over different cities for mosquito control, and farmers have used it to control insects. It is still in use today.

3.   Carbamates

    a.   These are similar to organophosphates but cause less permanent damage. They are being used as fungicides and herbicides. They are also used in clothing, medicines, and plastics. Symptoms such as blurred vision, weakness, memory loss, convulsions, and behavioral problems can occur for several hours after exposure. Other problems, such as thyroid function disturbance have also been reported.

Industrial Compounds and Chemical By-products —

Pesticides are not the only toxic chemicals to have infiltrated our environment. Man-made industrial compounds and their chemical by-products have also made a great impact on the world around us. What follows are a few of the major compounds that have achieved widespread integration into our day-to-day world.

1. Phthalates and Plasticizers

    a. Phthalates and plasticizers are found in industrial chemicals such as inks, adhesives, vinyl floor tiles, paints, and plastics such as plastic food wraps, plastic bottles, Styrofoam cups, plastic baby bottles, and plastic food containers. Phthalate from these plastic compounds can enter foods through direct contact, particularly during microwave heating, or when using plastic to wrap hot food.

    b. Bottled water in plastic containers can also be contaminated by these compounds when stored in a heated environment, such as a garage or car. Do not heat frozen foods with plastic containers in the microwave. Do not drink bottled water if it has been sitting in a heated environment for a long time. Do not drink coffee or hot tea in Styrofoam cups. Do not use plastic containers for foods that have been heated. Avoid buying foods in plastic containers such as fruit juices, ketchup, milk, or beverages.

    c. We are exposed to plasticizers every day. They are so thoroughly integrated with the packaging of our foods and our environment that they filter through our body day in and day out. These chemicals interrupt our hormone systems, especially the thyroid and sex hormones. They may cause boys to be more feminine.[63] They may also cause precocious puberty (early onset of puberty) in girls. Their long-term effects have yet to be seen, but I truly believe this is one of the major reasons for the increased cancer rate in the reproductive systems, such as breast and prostate cancers.

2. Solvents

    a. Solvents such as benzene, toluene, and xylene are commonly used as cleaning agents and a precursor to the manufacture of dyes, drugs, synthetic rubbers, and plastic products. These solvents are frequently labeled as "inert" and are not listed as ingredients in products, even though they may cause cancer and other serious diseases.

b.   Benzene is a universal solvent used in engine fuels and in the plastics, paint, and textile industries. It may damage bone marrow and thus lead to leukemia. Toluene is used to dissolve many common products, especially ink. Xylene is used in spray paints, plastics, photography, and in the leather and rubber industries. Both toluene and xylene can damage the nervous system, liver, kidneys, eyes, and skin.

Heavy Metals —

Heavy metals in our environment can also pose a threat to our health. Heavy metals are not biodegradable and hence accumulate in the environment. They enter the body through our air, water, and food. Once inside our bodies they accumulate in our fatty tissues, central nervous system, and bones. Heavy metals in general inactivate our enzyme systems, increase the production of free radicals, and damage mitochondria in the cells. They cause diseases so slowly that it is hard to recognize their impact or to even diagnose until late in the disease process.

1.   Mercury

a.   There is no safe level of mercury for humans. It is among the most toxic substances on the planet, right behind radioactive substances.

b.   Most people are exposed to mercury through dental amalgam, so-called "silver" fillings, which are composed of 50 percent mercury.

c.   Mercury vapors are continuously released from amalgam fillings, especially when eating foods with high temperature.

d.   Most fish are contaminated with mercury due to the polluted waters of their environment. According to the EPA, fish containing the highest levels of mercury are tuna, swordfish, mackerel, shark, halibut, ahi, snapper, and lobster. Fish with medium levels of mercury include sea bass, crab, and flounder. Fish with low levels of mercury are salmon, scallops, and shrimp.

e. Other sources of mercury come from additives in cosmetics, thimerosal (preservatives used in vaccines), latex paints, floor waxes, wood preservatives, and various batteries. Mercury is the most dangerous of all heavy metals. It interferes with mitochondrial function and thus with energy production.[64] Mercury increases oxidative stress and inflammation, as well as damages blood vessel walls and the immune system.[65] Mercury interferes with the liver detoxification pathways. It is a silent killer that cause diseases years after accumulated exposure. The symptoms of mercury toxicity are very nonspecific and, much like those exemplified by Mary's story, may just be fatigue or low immunity.

f. The dangers of mercury in the body are well known to the medical community. Clinically, mercury toxicity has been linked to many diseases that affect crucial body systems:

i. The Central Nervous System

1. This is the principle target organ.[66] Some of the diseases of the central nervous system that have been associated with mercury toxicity include:

a. Autism
b. Parkinson's disease
c. Tremor
d. Dementia and memory loss
e. Depression
f. Mental confusion or foggy mind
g. Neuropathy (numbness, tingling or weakness of extremities)

ii. The Cardiovascular System

1. Mercury toxicity can adversely affect the functioning of the cardiovascular system.

This is due to free radical damage to the vascular system, which causes atherosclerosis.[67] diseases associated with mercury toxicity are:

    a. Hypertension Cardio-vascular diseases

    b. Myocardial infarction (heart attack)

    c. Stroke

g. Autoimmune Disease or Lowered Immunity

    i. Our immune system, which is critical to keeping us healthy and protecting us from diseases, can be vulnerable to mercury toxicity, leading to conditions such as:

        1. Asthma

        2. Multiple sclerosis (MS)

        3. Frequent episodes of cold or flu

        4. Other Diseases

h. Mercury toxicity has also been linked to diseases such as:

    i. Chronic fatigue syndrome

    ii. Fibromyalgia

    iii. Multiple chemical sensitivities

    iv. Irritable bowel disease

    v. Cancer

Diagnosis for Mercury Poisoning

There are several ways to determine if your body is suffering from mercury poisoning.

1. History: If you have had multiple dental cavities with amalgam fillings for many years, or if you eat fish more than three times a week, you probably have too much mercury in your body.

2. Hair analysis: Testing strands of hair for heavy metals is an easy but not always accurate way to determine mercury levels, as hair only represents recent exposure.

3. Blood levels: If you have high or on-going exposure to mercury then your blood mercury levels will be elevated.

4.   RBC (red blood cells) mineral and heavy metals: This is a test that shows mercury in the tissue, but again it is limited to recent exposure as a RBC has only a ninety day life span. Watching mineral levels — especially zinc, selenium, and magnesium — is important because IV chelating may reduce them. When this occurs, these minerals must be replaced.

5.   Urine heavy metals: The most accurate test is the urine provocative test. This involves using DMSA (2, 3-dimercaptosuccinic acid) or DMPS (2, 3-dimercapto-1-propanesulfonic acid) orally or intravenously and collecting the urine for six hours afterwards. This test not only detects mercury, but a number of other heavy metals such as lead, cadmium, and arsenic. DMSA or DMPS are called chelators due to the fact that they act like a claw, grabbing mercury and other metals as they bring them from the liver through our detoxification systems, where they are eventually excreted in the urine and stool. It is a diagnostic as well as a therapeutic treatment.

Treatment for Mercury Poisoning

If your doctor has determined that you suffer from high levels of mercury exposure, then there a number of ways to help detoxify your system.

•   Remove the source of exposure. If you have amalgam fillings, you need to have them removed. It is always wise to take precautions if you decide to remove dental amalgams because you will be exposed to more mercury vapors in the process. The process for amalgam removal should only be done by dentists who are aware of the best way to prevent additional exposure to this toxic metal.

   o   Sometimes it is wise to remove only a few amalgam fillings at a time rather than many of them all at once, since the fewer that are removed the less the likelihood of heavy exposure to mercury. In order to help reduce exposure of the body to mercury during the amalgam removal process, IV chelation before and after the removal of silver fillings should also be planned.

o   If you have been eating fish or seafood known to have high mercury contamination, you need to reduce the amount you eat and replace them with fish that have less mercury exposure.

- Chelation with DMSA orally or DMPS intravenously. This is the most effective treatment method, but the drawback is that chelators grab other minerals and metals too, including the ones we want to keep, such as zinc, magnesium and selenium. It is important to assess and replace these minerals before and during chelation treatments.

o   It is important to check for any deficiencies in minerals and fatty acids and be sure to replenish them before beginning treatment. Without careful attention during this process, moving these nasty heavy metals can make you sicker.

- Oral chelation with amino acids which increase glutathion in our system can help the liver detoxify heavy metals including mercury. High dose magnesium, zinc and selenium compete and replace mercury which can reduce the mercury toxicity. Herbs such as cilantro detoxify mercury also. I recommend this form of treatment for my patients who are already sick from mercury poisoning.

2. Lead

a.   Like mercury, lead is a naturally occurring heavy metal that is recognized as an environmental health risk throughout the world. Although the ill-effects of lead toxicity have been recognized for thousands of years, it is still a ubiquitous metal that is used in everything from mining and refining to electrical wiring, paints, and ceramics. Some of the negative effects that lead poisoning can have on the body include:

i.   Anemia. Lead kills red blood cells by blocking their metabolism, which causes anemia.

  ii. Lead impairs development of the nervous system, which leads to learning disabilities, attention span deficits, and other behavioral problems in children.

  iii. Lead interferes with detoxification enzymes, causing oxidative stress, and cell death.

  iv. Houses built before 1978 can have lead paint and lead plumbing. Other sources of lead exposure include toys, ceramics with lead in the glaze, costume jewelry, leaded gasoline, fishing weights, bullets, and many others.

  v. After lead is absorbed in the body, it is deposited in the bones. When calcium leaks out of the bone at the time of a fracture or due to osteoporosis, lead seeps out as well. Acute lead poisoning is rare now but chronic, low level exposure still exists for children and adults. The tests used to detect mercury poisoning can also detect lead and other heavy metals. Hair analysis, blood and urine samples are all useful, especially following a DMSA or EDTA provocation test. Lead can be chelated out of the body much more easily than mercury. Sometimes the use of supplements consisting of 2,000 mg of vitamin C, 50 mg of B6, and 1,500 mg of calcium can eliminate lead from body tissues. IV chelation with EDTA and DMPS are approved treatments for lead poisoning.

3. Aluminum

  a. Aluminum is found in antacids, antiperspirants, pots and pans, aluminum foil, and baking powder. Aluminum is a bio-chemical that can attach to the phosphates in our DNA.[68] Once it binds with our DNA, the body cannot chelate it out by IV treatments. Excretion is mostly through the feces. There is no proven method for detoxifying aluminum, so avoidance is the best strategy. Avoid aluminum containing antiperspirants, antacids, aluminum canned foods, and cookware made of aluminum. Keep aluminum foil out of direct contact with food.

Sources of Chemicals in the Environment

The environment we live in today has changed quite a bit from the environment our parents and grandparents lived in. Today, toxic chemicals abound in our food, air and water supply. What follows is a brief listing of some of the most prevalent places such toxins can be found.

1. Foods
   a. Pesticides in our fruits and vegetables
   b. Hormones in animal meat, eggs, milk, and cheese Mercury in fish and other seafood
   c. Plasticizers in plastic food wraps, bottles, and containers
   d. Aluminum in aluminum food wraps
   e. Processed foods contain preservatives, sweeteners, MSG, and artificial food colors

2. Water
   a. Our water is home to a number of unhealthy chemicals, including fluoride, chloride, plasticizers, and chemical contaminants.

3. Air
   a. Chemicals contaminants can come from sources such as perfumes, car exhaust, gasoline and diesel fumes, sprayed pesticides, cleaning solutions, and paint.

4. Medical and Dental Treatments
   a. Certain treatments, such as vaccinations with thimerosal (ethyl mercury) and dental amalgam mercury fillings are toxic to the human body.

5. Skin Contact

    a.   Our skin can also absorb toxic contaminants through everyday household items, including:

        i.   Laundry detergents

        ii.   Cosmetics

        iii. Shampoos and hair dyes

        iv. Cleaning solutions

Our environment contains a large number of pollutants and chemicals toxins that exist in our homes and items we encounter each day, such as

- Lawn chemicals
- Building materials
- Carpet
- Paints
- Wood preservatives
- Leather treated with chemicals
- Clothing, especially dry cleaned garments
- Playgrounds and schoolyards sprayed with pesticides
- Flea soaps or pest collars for pets

Toxin Avoidance — How to Avoid Exposure to Toxins

The following tips will help you take positive steps towards detoxifying your diet and household environment:

- Always buy organic fruits, vegetables, and meat
- Eat foods in their natural form, not processed
- Stop eating fish and other seafood that contain high levels of mercury
- Remove mercury-based amalgam dental fillings
- Drink water filtered by a process of reverse osmosis or purified by a multi stage carbon filter
- Do not heat foods in plastic containers in microwave ovens

- Do not use plastic food wrap
- Use HEPA air filters or ionizers to reduce dust, molds and other indoor pollution
- Avoid using chemicals to clean your house. Use soap, baking soda, or vinegar instead
- Do not use pesticides in your lawn, garden, or house
- Use natural products for shampoos, cleaning solutions, hair dyes, and cosmetics
- Avoid products that contain aluminum, such as antiperspirants, antacids, as well as pots and pans
- Keep plenty of house plants to help filter indoor air
- Do not dry clean your clothes routinely. Be sure to air out dry cleaned clothes before wearing them
- If you smell anything putrid or acrid, try to clean the source of the smell right away. If this is not possible, try to put a comfortable distance between yourself and the source of the air pollution

How the Body Detoxifies

Just how does our body handle all of the environmental toxins that surround us and assault our internal systems each and every day? The answer involves a bit of biology, but it is actually quite interesting and easy to understand if we focus on the five main pathways of elimination in the body: the liver, gall bladder, kidneys, lymphatic system, colon, and sweat.

Detoxification is the process of the body's biochemical actions to eliminate unwanted chemicals. This process is mainly governed by the liver, which packages the unwanted chemicals to make them less toxic. The packaged chemicals then travel from the liver into the bile and are discharged into the intestines to be removed as feces.

Another route of excreting packaged chemicals is by traveling through the blood stream to the kidneys. Heavy metals and toxic chemicals are then excreted in the urine. Some toxins, especially heavy metals, migrate out of the body through the hair and nails. Another exit pathway for toxins is through perspiration and sweat.

The detoxification system helps the body eliminate excessive hormones and a wide variety of toxic chemicals such as drugs, heavy metals, pesticides and plastics. If the body does not detoxify well or is exposed to too many toxins, the toxic chemicals will deposit in the body's tissues and organs, especially in the central nervous and immune systems. These then form the underlying, or root cause of many diseases in the body.

1.   The Liver Pathway of Elimination

    a.   Detoxification starts at the liver, which is the most important detoxification organ in the body. There are two phases of detoxification in the liver.

        i.   Phase I

            1.   Phase I involves many protein enzymes, called cytochrome P450 enzymes. The chemical reaction involved is hydroxylation. Phase I produces many free radicals that can harm the body. It is like a waste treatment plant where more toxic intermediate products are produced. The nutrients used at Phase I are:

                a.   Riboflavin (vitamin A)
                b.   Niacin (vitamin B3)
                c.   Pyridoxine (vitamin B6)
                d.   Folic acid
                e.   Vitamin B12
                f.   Glutathione
                g.   Branch-chained amino acids
                h.   Flavonoids
                i.   Phospholipids

        ii.   Phase II

            1.   Phase II detoxification involves conjugation reactions, usually methylation and glucuronization. The Phase II detoxification pathway becomes very important to remove the more toxic intermediate products from Phase I. Lots of antioxidants are needed to reduce the

free radicals produced from the Phase I detoxification pathway.

2. Antioxidants to reduce free radicals at this stage are:

    a. Vitamin A
    b. Vitamin C
    c. Vitamin E
    d. Selenium Copper
    e. Zinc Manganese
    f. Coenzyme Q10 (Co-Q10)
    g. Bioflavonoids
    h. Milk thistle
    i. Pycnogenol
    j. Thiols (found in garlic, onions, and cruciferous vegetables such as broccoli and cauliflower)

3. Nutrients involved in the Phase II pathway are similar to the ones in Phase I, but additionally this phase requires a large amount of amino acids, such as:

    a. Glycine Taurine Glutamine
    b. N-acetylcysteine
    c. Cysteine Methionine

4. If we want to help the liver to detoxify, it is imperative to take the vitamins, minerals, and amino acids involved in the Phase I and II pathways.

Many enzymes are involved in the liver detoxification pathway, and these enzymes are related to our genetic makeup. For instance many Asians, including myself, are alcohol intolerant. On one occasion, I drank a Mai Tai thinking it was a non-alcoholic tropical drink. Within half an hour, my face began to flush; I had palpitations and felt very dizzy. These symptoms occurred because I do not have a powerful form of the enzyme acetaldehyde dehydrogenase. After the intestinal absorption of alcohol, it goes straight to the liver where the detoxification process starts. An enzyme called alcohol dehydrogenase converts the alcohol into acetaldehyde, which is thirty times stronger than alcohol. Then the enzyme acetaldehyde dehydrogenase converts the acetaldehyde into acetate (which is converted into fat), carbon dioxide, and water by another enzyme. Many Asians have a genetic variation that results in the production of a less powerful acetaldehyde dehydrogenase. The result is that the effect of alcohol is thirty times stronger for us, since more acetaldehyde stays in our system.

While we are on the subject of detoxification, let us take a look at how our body detoxifies estrogen. Starting in the liver, a Phase I detox pathway involves hydroxylation (OH). The OH can be linked to the number 2, or 4, or 16 carbon. The 2-OH metabolite becomes a weak estrogen, while the 4-OH and 16-OH metabolites still have a persistent estrogenic effect. This is important, because women who metabolize a larger proportion of their estrogen via the C-2 hydroxylation pathway tend to have a lower breast cancer rate compared to women who metabolize through the C-16 pathway. Which enzymatic route a woman metabolizes through is due to her own genetic variation. However, a diet high in cruciferous vegetables (i.e., broccoli, cabbage, and Brussels sprouts) can increase the C-2 hydroxylation pathway, which could reduce the risk of breast cancer.

After hydroxylation, the estrogen metabolites are oxidized to quinones, which become much more toxic to our body. This is the time when the Phase II detox pathway starts. The Phase II pathway involves methylation and glucuronization of the estrogen. The resulting metabolites are then excreted through the feces and urine.

Methylation requires B6, B12, folate, and magnesium, so a lack of these nutrients would slow down the detoxification of estrogen. Additionally, the presence of harmful intestinal bacteria can further complicate successful detoxification. Many of the most harmful bacteria have an enzyme called betaglucuronidase, which can uncouple the glucuronized estrogen and result in the estrogen being sent back to the liver to be detoxified again. Taking probiotics, such as acidophilus, will inhibit the harmful bacteria.

As a result of genetic variations leading to differences in detoxification enzymes, certain people can handle more toxic loads, while others become ill. If you do not have a good genetic make-up and do not have enough antioxidants and amino acids to help the enzymes in the detoxification pathways, you will begin to develop health problems if your toxic load is too high. Even a healthy individual with good genes and adequate nutrients runs the risk of developing diseases if their exposure to toxic chemicals is prolonged enough.

There are many ways to aid in the detoxification of your liver. Please remember to always consult with your physician first before embarking on any program of this type. One of the simpler ways to detoxify your liver is to begin taking daily supplements involving liver phase I and II pathways, as mentioned previously in this book.

Some people have such strong blockage of the bile duct that they have developed what is commonly known as gall stones or sluggish bile flow. There is a popular method known as the "Gall Bladder Flush." This flush method involves magnesium to help dilate the bile duct and oils to help stimulate the gall bladder contraction and apple juice to soften the gall stones.

If you want to try this method please follow the directions exactly as printed. Please note that this method may make you ill, nauseas and possibly vomit, so it is not to be done on a whim. Some patients have reported strong feelings of nausea lasting all day.

Here are the directions:

1. Drink one liter of diluted organic unsweetened apple juice daily for five days. During these 5 days eat raw organic fruits and vegetables. Avoid diary, meat and fried foods. Be certain you have bowel movements once or twice per day.

2. On the sixth day do not eat dinner and instead take one tablespoon of Epsom salts or 2000mg of magnesium at 6:00 p.m. with three glasses of water.

3. At 8:00 p.m. make a drink of 115 ml olive oil and 115 ml freshly squeezed citrus fruits such as grapefruit, orange, or lemon. Shake well and drink immediately.

4. The next morning you should pass green stones varying in sizes.

If you have a history of gall stones please consult your physician before trying this. You may need a longer preparation time and a higher dose of magnesium to accommodate the physical changes you will experience. I tried this flush myself and was surprised at the outcome. It was not an easy experience and required an entire day off as the feelings of nausea were strong, and I felt weak most of the day.

2.   The Kidney Pathway of Elimination

    a.   Our kidneys each contain about one million glomeruli, which are small balls of tiny blood vessels called capillaries. The capillary walls have many extremely tiny holes, which allow particles smaller than the holes to be filtered out of the capillaries into the urinary tract system, while keeping larger particles from escaping. The most common particles that are filtered out are actually water molecules, and more than 90 percent must be reabsorbed back into the capillaries to avoid dehydration. Toxins are filtered out this way, they are not reabsorbed.

    b.   To facilitate the excretion of toxins it is important to drink a lot of water. It is recommended that you drink 50 percent of your body weight in ounces. For example, if you weigh 150 pounds, then you should drink seventy-five ounces of water daily. One glass of water is about eight ounces.

3.   The Lymphatic System Pathway of Elimination

    a.   The lymphatic system is made of lymph nodes, ducts, tissues, and capillaries connected throughout the body. It is not as structured as the circulation system, which is an enclosed system that has a central pump (the heart). Rather, movement in the lymph system occurs with the milking action of the skeletal muscles when they move (contract), especially near the joints.

    b.   Toxins in the body's tissues can be transported to the lymphatic system by exercise or massage, and then excreted as sweat. The lymphatic system can also move the toxins into the circulatory system, where they are excreted in the urine. Exercise helps the body to detoxify by increasing blood circulation and lymphatic drainage.

    c.   I love to get massage regularly, knowing it not only relax me but also help my body to detox. I also do self-massage when I take my bath, It's really easy; just putting your fingers in your scalp, massage down to the neck area, along the side of the body, then down to the lower leg then to the feet.

4.   The Colon Pathway of Elimination

a.   The colon is the body's disposal system. It serves as a temporary holding tank for what the stomach and small intestine did not digest. It is also the normal residing place for more than 400 different kinds of bacteria. The most well-known bacteria are Lacto-bacillus acidophilus and Bifidobacteria, so-called friendly bacteria or probiotics.

b.   Unfortunately, some unfriendly bacteria and yeast also live in the GI (gastrointestinal) tract. Both of these organisms produce many toxins. In such situations, dysbiosis (abnormal bowel germ population) occurs. The harmful yeast or bacteria must be removed or reduced, and probiotics need to be reintroduced to accomplish this.

c.   We should have bowel movements once or twice a day. Constipation slows down the transit time of stool, allowing some of the toxins to be reabsorbed into the body. Chronic constipation means the body is not able to detoxify efficiently.

d.   To assist with moving digested food and eliminated toxins through the intestines, we need twenty to thirty grams of fiber daily. Fiber is the food source of healthy intestinal bacteria. It also prevents constipation.

e.   Good sources of fibers are:

i.   Flax seed. You can grind these small seeds in a coffee grinder, add the whole seed in your smoothie or buy them already ground.

ii.   Psyllium. The husk of the psyllium seed forms mucilage that absorbs excess water while stimulating normal bowel elimination.

    f.   Foods that are excellent sources of fiber include:

       i.   Leafy vegetables: cabbage, lettuce, and spinach.

      ii.   Stem and squash vegetables: broccoli, cauliflower, asparagus, and celery.

    iii.   Roots: carrots, beets, and turnips.

    iv.   Beans and legumes: green beans, soybeans, lentils, pinto, black, red, and yellow beans.

     v.   Grains: millet, rye, barley, and wild rice.

    g.   An increased intake of water and oils will help to reduce constipation. Exercise and intestinal massage also help. Avoid the long term use of laxatives that stimulate the bowels, such as Senekot or Peri Colace. The body eventually forms a dependence on these stimulants.

Colon hydrotherapy has been used as a method to clean out old stools, which accumulates in the mucosal folds of the colon. The use of colon hydrotherapy can be traced back 2,000 years and is still popular today.

    5.   The Sweat Pathway of Elimination

    a.   Another way the body eliminates toxins is through perspiration. Saunas developed by the Finns and sweat lodges used by Native Americans are good examples of the ways that people recognized the health benefits of sweating. A combination of exercise, vitamins, good nutrition, and regular use of the sauna can dislodge toxins from fatty tissues so that they can then be eliminated from the body by sweating.

    b.   If you have access to a sauna in a health club, do aerobic exercise first, take a shower and then sit in the sauna until you sweat. You can take a cold shower and go into the sauna again. Exposure to hot and cold will make the blood vessels dilate and constrict, which helps facilitate the excretion of toxins. If you have an infrared sauna at home, set the temperature from 120° to 140° F and sit in the sauna for twenty to thirty minutes. This will make you sweat profusely. Make sure you drink plenty water to replace the fluid you lose. Combined with exercise and a cold shower, it is a wonderful way to detoxify the body. The difference between an infrared sauna and a health club sauna is that the temperature in an infrared sauna can be adjusted to a lower degree so you can sit there longer, thereby sweating more toxins out of the body.

c.   Finding time to combine your sauna detoxification routine with other daily tasks can be easy and relaxing. I have an infrared sauna at home. I usually bring a book to read, an iPod for my favorite music, a jar of water and a big towel. I set the temperature to 125° F, and after thirty minutes I start to sweat profusely — I can even feel my heart starting to pound faster. When I feel that the sauna has become too hot I will turn it off, but will continue to remain inside for another ten to fifteen minutes and continue to sweat. This is one of my favorite activities and I get my reading done, toxins sweated out, muscles relaxed, and even get a cardio work out too by increasing my heart rate and all within forty-five minutes!

d.   Basic Detoxification — Points to Remember

   i.   Be aware that we live in a toxic world.

   ii.   Make sure toxin avoidance is part of your daily life.

   iii. Drink six to eight glasses of water daily.

   iv.   Have one or two bowel movements daily.

   v.   Sweat regularly by exercising or using a sauna.

   vi.   Regular exercise or lymphatic massage will improve lymphatic flow to help eliminate toxins.

   vii. Increase your fiber intake by eating more whole grains, nuts, seeds, and vegetables. Supplementation with flax seed or psyllium is helpful.

viii. Eat high-quality protein, such as eggs or whey protein, to help liver detoxification.

ix. Eat at least a cup of cruciferous vegetables (i.e., cabbage, broccoli, kale, cauliflower, Brussels sprouts) daily.

x. Eat celery, onions, grapes, berries, and citrus fruits to help the detoxification process.

xi. Use herbs such as cilantro, garlic, ginger, rosemary, turmeric, and curry for detoxification and anti-inflammation actions.

xii. Basic supplement for detoxification:

    1. High-potency multiple vitamin and mineral formula

        a. Vitamin C (1,000 mg daily)

        b. Milk thistle (100-200 mg daily)

        c. Omega-3 fatty acids (1,000-2,000 mg daily)

        d. Amino acids from whey or egg protein powder (2-4 tablespoons daily)

        e. Fiber, psyllium or flaxseed fiber (1-2 tablespoons with 8-16 ounces of water daily)

Electromagnetic Frequency (EMF) Contamination

Another potent source of environmental pollution originates from the electromagnetic fields generated by cell phones, power lines, wireless computers, and other electrical devices. Whenever electricity is used or generated, invisible lines of electric and magnetic force are created around its point of origin. Recent studies have raised concerns about the health effects of these electromagnetic frequencies, especially under prolonged exposure. The rapid growth of consumer electronics like cell phones and personal computers have brought the issue of EMF exposure to national attention, and an ever increasing number of national health organizations are recommending caution when it comes to the use of electric devices. To understand the effects of electromagnetic fields on the body, let us take a look at the relationship between electricity and the body's cellular functions.

The body generates its own electricity. That is why we can do an EKG (electrocardiogram) to check a person's heartbeat and an EEG (electroencephalogram) to check their brain waves. Chinese medicine has long called this bio-electricity Chi, our own energy pathway.

When we turn on a light, electricity passes through the wires powering it. The flow of electrons in this circuit creates a magnetic field. When we turn off the light, the flow of electrons ceases and the magnetic field disappears. The greater the light's power, the stronger the magnetic field it creates.

The body will only conduct electricity if the electrical field is strong enough. However, external magnetic fields or electromagnetic frequencies (EMF), such as those generated by electrical systems used to power homes and buildings, can penetrate the body without our awareness whenever we are within reach of that magnetic field. If the energy field is affected by this exposure to EMF, cellular functions may also be affected.

We are exposed to EMF contamination from the environment, workplace, and home appliances. Here are some helpful tips and strategies you can employ to help minimize your exposure to EMFs:

- Homes, playgrounds, and schools should be at least 350 feet from high- voltage transmission lines and at least fifty feet from pole mounted step-down transformers.

- A portable hair dryer can generate high EMF. Keep it away from your head. Wall-mounted hair dryers found in hotels are safer.

- The appliances in kitchens, such as refrigerators, microwaves, electric ovens, dishwashers, juicers, blenders, coffee makers, and toasters can have cumulative effects on EMF. Keep three feet away from these appliances, if possible.

- TVs, CD and DVD players, radios, computers, and printers generate EMF. Keep three feet away, if possible.

- Lights and alarm clocks in the bedroom generate EMF. Keep them at least five feet away from your head.

- Cell phones generate microwaves, just like a microwave oven does. Data concerning the health effects of cell phone-generated microwaves are mounting, but there is currently no consensus on how safe they are. Avoid using your cell phone for an extended period of time. For safety, avoid using your cell phone while you are driving.

Multiple Chemical Sensitivities

Given the large amount of toxic substances in our environment, it is no wonder that many people develop sensitivities and allergies to a number of different chemicals. Yet despite its growing prevalence, this condition is not something that many people are aware of.

Multiple Chemical Sensitivity can best be thought of in this way: imagine that your waste management company has gone on strike, and that garbage has begun to accumulate in your house. The longer the strike, the more the garbage accumulates. The more garbage in your house, the more smelly and dirty your house gets.

It does not matter whether we are exposed to a large amount of toxins all at once, as migrant agricultural workers are with pesticides, or if our bodies accrue small amounts of toxins over an extended period of time due to factors like poor nutrition or mercury leaking from dental fillings. Once we have enough toxins accumulated in the body, we become sick. Not everyone is affected in the same way because of our genetic differences. These differences affect our capacity to detoxify from chemical substances. Symptoms vary from person to person also, with the most common target organ being the brain. The symptoms of chemical sensitivity can range from fatigue, joint pain, mood swings, brain fog, headaches, dizzy spells, and nausea or flu like illness. Individuals become sensitive and allergic to almost everything. Poor diet, stressful situations, and a lack of sleep and exercise certainly make things worse.

Patients who develop multiple chemical sensitivities usually undergo a battery of tests and try multiple medications, only to find that the tests yield no definitive results and the medications make their symptoms worse. It is frustrating for physicians, but even more so for the patients themselves who are tired of being told, "It's all in your head."

There is no standard test physicians can order to confirm the diagnosis. To make things even more confusing, the patients may present multiple symptoms and diagnoses such as fibromyalgia, chronic fatigue syndrome, hypochondria, neurosis, irritable bowel syndrome, chronic insomnia, migraine headaches, neurodegenerative diseases, asthma, hay fever, and auto immune diseases. Many of them have leaky gut syndrome, which opens the gate for toxins getting into our body through the GI tract.

However, there are some tests that may be helpful in determining Multiple Chemical Sensitivities:

- A RBC toxic metal and mineral screen.
- A urine challenge test with DMPS.
- A food allergy test.
- A comprehensive stool analysis.
- Antibodies for Candida or wheat.

The treatments are individualized but generally include:

- Toxin avoidance: clean air, clean water, clean house, and clean food.
- Improving nutritional status: avoiding foods the patient is allergic to and replacing healthy bacteria to improve the GI defense mechanism.
- Detoxification with general detox supplements.
- Specific treatments such as IV or oral DMPS chelation for mercury, as well as IV treatments with high doses of the vitamins and minerals that are involved in the liver Phase I and II pathways.

There is no question that we live in a changing environment. The amount of industrial, chemical, and other artificial pollutants contaminating our air, water, and food supply has never been higher, so much so that it is no longer a question of whether we have toxins in our body or not, but how much we can limit the damage that is being done.

Even in our toxic world it is still possible to experience optimal health and reap the maximum benefit from healing treatments such as bio-identical hormone therapy by reducing our exposure to environmental toxins. Taking positive steps to rid our households of toxic chemicals, improve our nutritional status, and detoxify periodically can make the difference between merely functioning day-to-day and thriving with physical energy, mental clarity, and zest for life!

Chapter 12

How to Look 10 Years Younger — Beauty Is Not Just Skin Deep

The Skin

The skin is the largest organ of the body. There are approximately nineteen million skin cells on every square inch of the body and the skin keeps renewing itself throughout our lifetime. The primary function of the skin is protection. The skin provides an elastic and waterproof covering to the body to protect it from germs, heat, cold, and the damaging effects of ultraviolet rays in sunlight. The skin has three layers: the epidermis, dermis, and subcutaneous layer.

Skin Structure

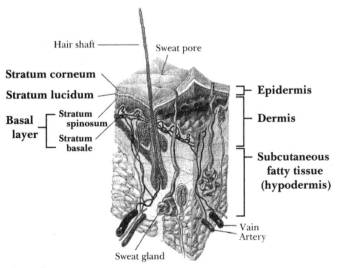

Figure 7.

Epidermis, Outer Layer

The epidermis has five layers that form the outermost layer of the skin. These layers work together to continually replenish the epidermis in order to form a supple, healthy covering for the body.

1. Stratum corneum: external layer of the epidermis that holds water inside the body and prevents the entrance of ultraviolet light, pollutants, and chemicals into the body. It is constantly shedding and replenishing itself, completely replacing this layer every month. This process slows down as we get older. Helping this layer shed by using a loofah or body brush will help keep the skin looking younger by removing dead skin cells from the surface.

2. Stratum lucidum (clear layer): second layer of the epidermis that consists of small, transparent cells. When the outer layer of cells on the stratum corneum sheds, this layer moves up to become the top layer of the epidermis, which turns over constantly.

3. Stratum granulosum: exists only in the thick skin found in the palms of the hands and soles of the feet. It helps form a tougher, waterproof barrier to the skin in these areas.

4. Stratum spinosum: also exists only in the thick skin areas of the body. It provides structural support to help the skin resist abrasion.

5. Stratum basale: the third layer (fifth layer in hands and feet) of the epidermis generates new epidermal skin cells that will eventually move outward, layer by layer, to become the outermost layer. This deepest layer of the epidermis also contains melanocytes, which produce melanin, a pigment that protects the skin from excessive damage resulting from ultraviolet light. Darker skin results from the production of more melanin. Caucasians have fewer melanocytes, compared to Asians or Africans, which accounts for their lighter skin tone.

Unfortunately, this lack of melanin means there is less protection to the skin from sun damage. Overexposure to ultraviolet sunlight leads to skin cancer and wrinkles. With aging, damaged melanocytes join together, forming pigment blotches that are called sun spots. Malignant melanoma is a cancer of the melanocytes.

Dermis: The Middle Layer

Lying beneath the epidermis, the skin's middle layer is composed of collagen, elastin, and hyaluronic acid, the latter of which holds water. Also embedded in the dermis are blood vessels, lymph vessels, nerve endings, sweat glands, oil glands, and hair follicles.

As skin ages, it loses collagen and elastin. As the body's hormone levels decrease with aging, less oil production occurs for feeding the collagen and elastin. Also with aging, less water retention within the cells results in reduced hyaluronic acid. Both of these impairments lead to the wrinkles that develop in the skin.

Subcutaneous: The Inner Layer

This layer is mainly composed of fat, plus the blood vessels, lymph vessels, and nerves that feed into the dermis. The body loses subcutaneous fat as we age, mostly due to a decline of hormones. This causes the deeper wrinkles, sagging and thinning of the skin.

Skin Damage

The most damaging factor to the skin results from overexposure to sunlight. Other deleterious factors are free radicals that occur as a result of exposure to cigarette smoke, pollutants, harmful bacteria, chemicals, and toxins.

Sun damage causes the skin to develop pigmented blotches; it loses its elasticity and collagen, leading to sun spots, wrinkles and saggy skin. If you look at your inner arm versus the side exposed to the sun, you will find that the differences in appearance are all due to sun damage.

The sun's electromagnetic radiation generates three types of ultraviolet (UV) light:

1. UVA has the longest wave length and penetrates deeper into the skin layers. This causes tanning of the skin, but it also destroys collagen and elastin in the dermis. Indeed, this UVA light causes the most damage to the

skin, yet most tanning salons use this light. It is a slow-reacting light wave and it takes about an hour to get sunburned from exposure to this light.

2. UVB, the medium wave length, penetrates less into the skin compared to UVA, but it causes moderate tanning of the skin. It only takes twenty to thirty minutes for UVB to cause sunburn.

3. UVC the shortest wave and is rarely heard of because most UVC is filtered out by the earth's ozone layer, therefore exposure only occurs at high altitudes or in areas where the ozone layer is damaged (notably, Antarctica). This very short light wave does not penetrate into the skin deeply, but it can cause sunburn within just one minute of exposure.

Principles of Keeping Your Skin Youthful

Taking steps to protect and nourish your skin is an essential part of every anti-aging plan. Here are the primary rules you should observe in order to keep your skin looking healthy and vibrant for years to come.

- Avoid sun damage. Wear a large rim hat with SPF 30 or over. Apply sunscreen to exposed skin to protect yourself from both UVA and UVB. Avoid exposure to the sun between 10 A.M. and 3 P.M., when UV light is at its strongest. Most sunscreens have toxic chemicals that can enter into our body and cause inflammation and cellular damage. The only safe one to use is Zinc oxide, which does not penetrate our skin but leave a white layer on the skin. Try to use a product that has smaller molecules of Zinc, does not leave a white color on the skin and does not penetrate into the skin. Also using cream with antioxidants will neutralize the free radicals and further protect your skin. Be sure to frequently reapply them if you are exposed to the sun continuously or engaged in outdoor activities such as hiking, swimming, or gardening.

- Hydrate your skin. The easiest way to hydrate your skin is to drink plenty of water. Additionally, most moisturizers cover and seal your skin to prevent water loss. A mini-facial helps moisturize your skin, such as using a wet towel or steam on your face. Then while the water is still on your skin, seal it with oil such as vitamin E or coconut oil.

- Nourish your skin. Your skin needs nutrition just like any other part of the body. It is difficult to give nutrition to the skin through a topical cream because the epidermis is a natural barrier. Nonetheless, many capillaries circulate blood just beneath the epidermis, so it is important to get the nutrients that the skin needs through blood circulation. By eating a nutritious diet, you will help to ensure that your skin receives the nutrients it needs.

- Keep your hormones levels in the younger age range. Estrogen increases subcutaneous fat and connective tissue, thus it assists in the prevention of wrinkle formation. Testosterone increases the secretion of oil glands and prevents dryness of the skin.

Treatment for Pigmented Skin Blotches and Sun Spots

If your skin is already damaged due to aging and sun exposure, there are steps you can take to repair the damage and keep your skin looking great. In addition to these treatments, be sure to follow the principles for keeping your skin youthful, as discussed above, in order to help maintain your skin's health and appearance.

- Inhibit the formation of melanin (skin pigment) by using creams that contain hydroquinone, kojic acid, or herbs.

- Remove melanin by using Retin-A, skin peel, or laser treatment. Retin-A (or retinol) cream is a form of vitamin A that peels the skin and stimulates growth of the epidermis. Skin peels are usually performed by an aesthetician who applies different chemicals. The beneficial effect of this treatment is limited to the superficial epidermis layer. Laser or light therapy, such as IPL (intense pulsed light), removes deeper epidermal skin layers and also stimulates the formation of collagen.

- Protect new skin by reducing your exposure to the sun.
- Treatment for Wrinkles and Sagging Skin
- Wrinkles, fine lines and sagging skin resulting from aging and sun damage can also benefit from the following treatments.
- Increase your skin turnover (shedding and replacement of new skin) by using glycolic acid or Retin-A cream.
- Resurface the skin with a facial peel, laser treatment, or IPL (intense pulse light).
- Increase your collagen through laser or IPL treatment. Collagen injections can also help to improve suppleness and elasticity and give you immediate results.
- Botox injections may relax the muscles in the forehead and around the eyes, thus reducing the wrinkles in that area.

Laser and IPL

Laser and IPL (intense pulsed light) are light wave treatments for the skin. Different light has varying wave lengths, some of which can reach certain parts of the skin such as pigment layers, hair follicles or blood vessels. Laser has either ablative (removal) or partially ablative abilities. With laser treatment, the superficial layers of the skin can be totally or partially removed. IPL is not immediately ablative; therefore, the skin is not removed at the time of treatment. However, it does cause the skin to peel a few days later. Peeling of the old skin leads to newer and younger skin. Both treatments can be used to stimulate the formation of collagen and remove pigmented lesions or hairs. These treatments can be combined to achieve better results for skin rejuvenation. Partial skin ablation, such as Fraxel or Pixel Laser treatment, results in less down time for recovery than total skin ablation, such as CO_2 (carbon dioxide) laser or Erbium laser treatment. Partial skin ablation is safer; however, it requires a series of treatments rather than just one treatment. Nonetheless, this approach has grown in popularity since the down time is minimal following treatment.

The side effects of these treatments can be skin irritation; hypo-pigmentation (loss of skin color), and hyper-pigmentation, which causes patches of skin to become darker in color than the surrounding skin. Generally speaking, lighter skin types have fewer complications than individuals with darker skin because with lighter skin there is less pigmentation of skin cells.

After laser or IPL treatment, it is important to follow the recommended skin care program in order to maintain younger looking skin. Without such a maintenance program, the treated skin will return to its less than optimal condition.

Home Skin Care

Great skin care begins at home. In addition to minimizing your sun exposure and eating a balanced nutritious diet, try the following simple suggestions to supercharge your personal skin care program.

- Avoid sun damage. Use sunscreen with a minimal rating of SPF 15 that includes UVA and UVB protection. Apply each morning before leaving the house. Make sure your sunscreen has natural ingredients, not harsh chemicals, and that it also contains moisturizers and antioxidants. Also, mineral makeup powder has the effect of working as a sunscreen.

- Hydrate your skin at night by steaming your face or putting a wet towel on your face while bathing. Seal the moisture right afterward by massaging vitamin E oil on your face. Spraying your face with thermal spring water periodically throughout the day also helps.

- Use creams that have retinol or glycolic acid daily to stimulate the removal of old skin and the formation of new skin. This will also help the nutrients in the facial cream penetrate into the facial skin.

- Maintain youthful skin by using good skin care products to clean, hydrate, and nourish your skin twice a day. I recommend a total skin care system that consists of sun screen, antioxidant serum and retinal for skin repair regeneration. Regular use of these skin care products can reduce and reverse changes that come with aging skin, such as wrinkles, age spots, and thinning of the skin.

Do facial treatments regularly, administered either by an aesthetician or by yourself. Remember beauty is not just skin deep. Good nutrition and supplements, regular exercise, adequate sleep, stress reduction, maintaining your hormones in good range, and reducing toxin exposure are all very important in maintaining your beautiful and healthy skin!

Chapter 13

Our Mind — You Are What You Think

In this chapter, we are going to explore the science of the mind-body connection and the potential it has to help us heal in ways we would never have thought possible.

The Mind — Body Connection

Think of our body as a computer. If the brain is the hardware, the mind is the software. The brain controls the body through hormones and neurotransmitters; the mind governs the brain with thoughts and feelings. Together, they rule our behavior, emotions, and the many different functions of our body. Everything we do starts from the mind. It is extremely powerful, and it can make you or break you!

Let us look at how the mind exerts its influence. If you simply think, for example, of eating a lemon, without even seeing the lemon you start to secrete saliva just by thinking about how sour it is. Or if you receive a letter from the IRS (Internal Revenue Service), your mind races even before you have opened the letter as you wonder if the IRS plans to audit you. Your heart pounds a little faster and anxiety arises. After you open the letter and discover the IRS is going to refund you a few thousand dollars, your heart beat slows down again and you feel happy knowing that you will not be facing an ordeal.

It is estimated that over half of the office visits to family practitioners or general internists are due to emotionally related physical symptoms. If the physician focuses on the illness without paying attention to the underlying emotional cause then that illness will probably not improve much, and additional emotionally driven illnesses will probably also occur.

The Brain

The human brain has three parts: the forebrain, midbrain, and hindbrain. The fore brain contains lobes of the cerebral cortex that control higher functions, such as thinking, reasoning, and speaking. The midbrain and hindbrain control the unconscious autonomic functions of the body. Specific behaviors are associated with different parts of the brain.

- The Cerebrum
  - o The cerebrum, the evolutionary new part of the human brain, is divided into symmetric left and right hemispheres. Within these hemispheres are the prefrontal and frontal cortex, temporal lobes, basal ganglia, occipital lobes, hypothalamus, and the pituitary glands.
  - o The frontal lobes are divided into three parts:
    - The motor cortex, which controls movement such as walking.
    - The premotor cortex, which involves the planning of motor movement.
    - The prefrontal cortex, which coordinates planning, organization impulse control, and communication.
  - o The prefrontal cortex is the most evolved part of a human being. It is what makes humans stand out from other animals. This is the part of the brain from which anxiety and worry emanate.
  - o If this part of the brain works right, a person is organized, thoughtful, empathetic, and communicative. They can learn from mistakes and make plans to reach goals. When it does not work adequately it results in poor judgment, a short attention span, trouble learning from experience, poor time management, or difficulty with organization to perform tasks.

- o The temporal lobes lay at the sides of the brain and are involved with the subconscious mind. The functions carried on here are:
  - Short-term memory and memory storage
  - Language and auditory (hearing) processing
  - Storage of remembered feelings and emotions
- o Problems in the temporal lobes lead to memory loss, learning and reading difficulties, difficulty with speech, or unstable moods. This is the first area damaged by Alzheimer's disease.
- o The basal ganglia area is involved with:
  - Motor control
  - Cognition
  - Emotions
  - Learning
- o Low activity in this area, such as in patients with Parkinson's disease, leads to slow movement, tremors, and problems with writing, walking, and other daily activities.
- Other diagnoses linked to injured basal ganglia include, among others, ADHD (attention deficit hyperactivity disorder), cerebral palsy, obsessive-compulsive disorder, and stuttering.
- The occipital lobes are located in the back of the skull. It is the visual processing center where everything that we see is interpreted, analyzed, and integrated with the other parts of the brain.
- Hypothalamus and pituitary glands. The hypothalamus secretes hormones to regulate the pituitary gland. Located at the bottom of the brain, the pituitary gland hangs like a little pearl into its own small, protective skull pocket. It secretes growth hormone along with other hormones that control the thyroid and adrenal glands, as well as the ovaries or testes.
- The Cerebellum. The cerebellum, also called the small brain, is the older part of the brain. Even though its size

represents only 10 percent of the brain, it contains 50 percent of the brain's neurons or nerve cells. Located at the bottom of the brain, it is the major motor coordination center. Problems in this part of the brain result in poor handwriting, or being clumsy or accident-prone.

Neurotransmitters and the Neuroendocrine Communication System

Neurotransmitters are the chemical messengers that have either inhibitory or excitatory functions. If the neurotransmitters are balanced, the brain will be balanced. Too much stimulatory neurotransmitters or not enough inhibitory neurotransmitters will make a person nervous or anxious, while the opposite leads to depression or other problems.

There are six major neurotransmitters:

- Neuro-excitatory: epinephrine (adrenaline), norepinephrine, glutamate.

- Neuro-inhibitory: serotonin, GABA (gamma-aminobutyric acid).

- Both excitatory and inhibitory: dopamine.

Acetylcholine is another neurotransmitter that is typically involved with memory.

- Serotonin

   o Serotonin is the most well-known and studied neurotransmitter because many antidepressant medications, such as Prozac, Zoloft, and Paxil, are selective serotonin re-uptake inhibitors (SSRIs). This means that these medications increase the level of serotonin to relieve depression. All neurotransmitters are made from amino acids, so if the intake of the precursor amino acids is increased, neurotransmitters will also increase.

   o The amino acid tryptophan converts to 5 HTP (5-hydroxytryptophan), which then converts to serotonin. This neurotransmitter further converts to melatonin, which is the hormone that helps regulate sleep.

o   When serotonin is low, norepinephrine or dopamine may be over expressed, resulting in the fight-or-flight response and leading to panic attacks and anxiety. Low levels of serotonin lead to low melatonin, which causes insomnia. Low serotonin levels are also associated with PMS (premenstrual syndrome), eating disorders, migraine headaches, and depression.

- GABA

o   GABA (gamma-aminobutyric acid) is a neuro-inhibitory neurotransmitter. Low levels of GABA lead to insomnia, irritability, anxiety and panic attacks. Amino acids, such as theanine and taurine, increase the functions of GABA, as do tranquilizers and alcohol.

- Dopamine

o   Dopamine has both an inhibitory and excitatory function. It increases the secretion of growth hormone (GH) by increasing GH-releasing hormone, and plays a major role in motor function, memory, cognition, and focus.

o   Dopamine deficiency can result in attention deficit disorder (ADD), poor memory, and motor dysfunction, as seen in Parkinson's disease. Low levels of dopamine also mean low levels of pleasure. The SSRI (selective serotonin re-uptake inhibitor) group of antidepressants inhibits dopamine function, which helps to explain why people on antidepressants may have low libido, or be emotionally flat.

- Epinephrine, Norepinephrine, and Glutamate

o   Epinephrine, norepinephrine, and glutamate are all excitatory neurotransmitters. Epinephrine (adrenaline) is the principle hormone produced by the adrenal glands. It travels through the blood stream to the brain. Another source of epinephrine occurs from the conversion of norepinephrine in the presence of cortisol. These hormones have excitatory functions and have to be balanced with inhibitory neurotransmitters in order for individuals to function well.

Brain Health and Hormones

Hormones have a deep impact on the brain because they are essential players in the fundamental communication of billions of nerve cells. In their roles as regulators and stimulators, hormones are responsible for brain functions that determine mood status, memory storage, cognitive capacities and sexual desires. Let us take a look at each one of them:

- Estrogen
- Increases the amount of mood regulating neurotransmitters, including norepinephrine, serotonin, and also acetylcholine, which improves memory.
- Increases the density of neurotransmitter receptors on the cell membrane of neurons, which helps improve the functioning of the neurotransmitters.
- Increases the growth and survival of nerve cells. Estrogen deficiency may lead to brain atrophy and death of nerve cells.
- Increases the ability of neurons to connect in various part of the brain, regulating emotional states such as depression and anxiety.
- Is necessary for blood flow to the parts of brain that are responsible for emotion, memory and cognitive functions.
- Progesterone involved in mood and memory, but through a different pathway than estrogen may counterbalance and offset some of the effects of estrogen on mood and memory.

- o Increases GABA levels by converting to allopregnenolone, which is one of the most potent modulators of GABA receptors in brain cells. By increasing the calming neurotransmitter GABA, progesterone helps women relax and sleep better.

- **Testosterone**
  - o Influences the areas of brain that regulate sexual responsiveness.
  - o It increases libido and is a powerful treatment for sexual dysfunction in both men and women.
  - o Influences cognitive function, and improves both learning and memory.
  - o Improves the mood and can work as an effective antidepressant, without the side effects of antidepressant medications.

- **Thyroid Hormone**
  - o It is well known that depression can be the result of low thyroid hormone. Thyroid hormones regulate metabolism for the whole body and if thyroid hormones are low, nothing works right. Depression, irritability, memory loss and brain fog are common symptoms when thyroid is low.

- **Cortisol**
  - o Excessive cortisol (cortisone) inhibits serotonin through different mechanisms at receptor sites in brain cells. Cortisol also converts norepinephrine to epinephrine. When this happens, external stress can lead to increased anxiety or depression.

In summary, 5-HTP, thyroid hormone, estrogen and testosterone all boost serotonin function. Progesterone improves GABA levels. Estrogen and testosterone both improve acetylcholine levels, and the blood circulation to the brain, thus they improve memory and slow down brain aging.

With many of my patients I have been able to gradually reduce and then discontinue use of antidepressants once estradiol and/or testosterone pellet implants have begun to work. I also use bio-identical progesterone, either in the form of cream, lozenges, or pills in women who suffer from PMS, insomnia, anxiety, and moodiness with good results.

When we treat mood issues in menopausal women or andropausal men, hormone treatment should be the first choice, not antidepressants or tranquilizers. Reducing stress hormones and optimizing the thyroid hormone can also contribute significantly to the improvement of mood and cognitive functions of the brain.

The neuroendocrine system is very complex. It involves neurons, neurotransmitters, hormones, carrier proteins and receptors. Treatments that help balance neurotransmitters and hormones are the keys to optimal health.

How to Improve Brain Health

Brain cells, like other cells in the body, need balanced hormones, adequate nutrition and oxygen, as well as avoidance of exposure to toxins. Here are ways to help maintain good health for the brain:

- Brain cells do not repair as easily as cells in other organs. In fact, until recently, it was believed that brain cells could not even regenerate. Precautions should always be taken to minimize the risk of head injuries. Always wear a helmet when riding a bicycle or motorcycle.

- Aerobic exercise brings more blood to the brain, which results in more oxygen and nutrients.

- Specific brain exercises will build new transmission pathways and enhance brain function. Learning to do new things is a form of mental exercise. Music, dance, reading books, creative writing or doing crossword puzzles are all good examples of brain exercises.

- Balanced and optimized hormones such as estrogen, testosterone, progesterone, and thyroid hormones are very important for the brain to function well.

- Stress reduction is important because high levels of cortisol and adrenaline (epinephrine) interfere with brain function.

- A high protein and low-carbohydrate diet is essential for a healthy brain because neurotransmitters are made from amino acids, which are derived from protein. High or low levels of sugar will adversely affect the brain's capacity to work.

- Avoid stimulants like caffeine, as they worsen anxiety. Alcohol's depressive function on the brain also interferes with optimal brain health.

- Good fat, especially DHA (docosahexaenoic acid) from omega-3 fatty acids, is a building block for cell membranes of the brain. It also protects the brain by reducing inflammation.

- Supplements such as 5-HTP and SAMe (S-adenosyl-L-methionine) increase the body's level of serotonin. Melatonin helps with sleep. Many antioxidants help prevent brain aging.

The Conscious, Subconscious, and Unconscious Mind

The majority of the mind is unconscious, and is formed during the first few years of life. The conscious mind is just the tip of the iceberg. Between the conscious and unconscious levels of the mind is the subconscious, which can be brought to conscious awareness when an individual is deeply relaxed.

The unconscious mind is made of suppressed memories and remembered feelings from early childhood. Its impressions are established very early in life. These impressions are carried throughout a person's lifetime without that person knowing much about its content.

A person can have a panic attack, for example, and never know what brought on the feeling of dread that triggered the episode. Or someone can go into an uncontrollable rage in reaction to a very minute incident. Or an individual can be attracted to another person without really knowing why. Or a person cannot control eating habits, even though that person knows not to overeat.

These are examples of when we know at a conscious level that we should or should not do certain things, but mental blocks in the subconscious or unconscious hold us back.

The distinction between the unconscious level of mind and the subconscious is a fine line. We can access the subconscious mind when we reduce conscious control through meditation or hypnosis. We can screen our thoughts consciously in an attempt to figure out what the subconscious is telling us.

The mind is largely composed of the thoughts, feelings, sensations and behavioral feedback that emanate from all of its levels: the conscious, subconscious and unconscious. If we can better understand what is going on in the subconscious and unconscious levels, we can train our conscious mind to reduce negative thoughts and to develop positive thoughts instead. We can also tap into our subconscious mind for creativity and unleash the massive potential that is innate to our being. In other words, by working to integrate these three levels of the mind, the outcome can be wondrously improved. We do not have to stay stuck in patterns of thinking, feeling and behaving.

How does one tap into the subconscious, and open the hidden power of our mind? Meditation, creative visualization, positive affirmation and self-hypnosis are all important tools.

Meditation

Meditation is the act of letting your mind become quiet and removing noisy thoughts from your conscious level. As you relax and the mind becomes quiet, you will be able to connect to your subconscious. Meditation is one of the most important tools you have to tap into the treasures of your subconscious mind. Meditation can be performed in an extended session of 20 to 45 minutes, or a short session that can take less than five minutes.

Steps for Creative Visualization, Guided Imaginary and Positive Affirmations:

For those that have an active mind and find it difficult to calm your mind, creative visualization and affirmation are much easier to do. Try with a good relaxation CD and with guided imagery you will be on your way!

- Sit comfortably in a chair or on the floor or lie on a bed and close your eyes.

- Take a deep breath; inhale and exhale slowly; relax your body.

- Count down from fifty to one. Relax your body from head to toe progressively by first contracting and then relaxing the muscles in your neck, face, eyes and jaw. Then move gradually downward as you relax your shoulders, arms, hands, fingers, back, belly, and hips, moving further downward toward your thighs, calves, ankles, and, lastly, your feet and toes.

- Now that your body is relaxed, start the creative visualization and positive affirmations. Repeat them mentally. Here are examples of positive affirmations:
  o I am calm, I am relaxed.
  o I am confident, I am at peace.
  o I am kind, I am compassionate.
  o I am healthy, I am attractive.
  o I maintain a healthy body and mind.

Creative visualization, positive affirmations, and self-hypnosis are very similar. Combined with meditation, they can become powerful tools to reshape your mind and change your life. As little as ten minutes a day will do wonders if you are persistent! Here are some examples:

  o Visualize yourself playing tennis. You run smoothly, arriving just in time to accurately hit the ball with a crisp sound.

  o Visualize yourself giving a presentation. You walk into a room full of people, greet them, smile, and begin your presentation with confidence, calmness and articulate clarity.

  o Visualize the fat in your abdominal area melting away.

  o Visualize a laser gun destroying a tumor in your body.

  o Recall the sights, sounds and feelings associated with the memory. Remember any particular smells, the taste of certain foods and the touch of different objects and people.

o Imagine your goal has been achieved. Sense the sights, savor the sounds; Recall the smells and remember feelings that accompany this success.

o Visualize a golden ray of energy coming into your body through your feet, moving upward along your thighs, pelvis, stomach, heart and lungs, and brain. This golden light brings a flood of energy that is healing every part of your body.

Once we learn how to tap into our subconscious mind, the next step is to do an honest assessment of ourselves, our self-esteem and how to improve it. Developing people skills and learning how to relate to one another is also very important, as most problems we encounter in life start from relationship issues.

Self-esteem

Self-esteem is how we see and value ourselves subconsciously. Typically, this is the result of remembered feelings that have originated from childhood experiences that carry through to adulthood. It is the self-image formed as an individual internalizes feedback from the environment.

A person who was raised in a negative environment as a child and was constantly criticized or punished would predictably have low self-esteem, even if extremely intelligent. Worst of all, when that person grows up, the subconscious and unconscious will continue the pattern of criticism to which that person has become accustomed. Low self-esteem can lead to failure in school, work and social interactions. Past failures will further lower one's self-esteem, which will only lead to more failures in the present. This then becomes a vicious cycle of ongoing self-defeat.

Low self-esteem often leads to depression or anxiety, or both. It is also a major reason people do not reach their full potential. To build self-esteem, you need to do an honest evaluation of yourself, recognizing that everybody has strengths and weaknesses and establish goals and objectives to help create what you want.

Implanting positive thoughts and emotions through creative imagination and self-hypnosis are very effective ways to not only improve self-esteem but to help a person achieve their life ambitions. Be mindful of your thoughts and your emotions. Whenever you experience negative emotions such as anger, frustration, depression or anxiety, it is always due to the negative thoughts you have. Consciously change your thoughts to more positive thoughts. It is like pulling the weeds out and planting more flowers in the garden to make it a lovely place to enjoy.

Chapter 14

Spirit — Your True Power

Have you ever felt uplifted after meeting someone who is kind and loving, your spirit seems lifted and you feel happier? Have you noticed how much better you feel after climbing a mountain or walking by the ocean? Do you notice how your energy gets better and your mind becomes clearer after these experiences?

Anatomy of the spirit

Our body produces its own energy, more precisely, subtle energy. This energy system is what allows physicians to perform an EKG (electrocardiogram) to detect the activity of the heart, or EEG (electroencephalogram) to detect the activity of brain. This is what Chinese call "chi." According to quantum physics, life energy is not static, it is a vibration. We are electric magnetic beings.

I never quite understood what spirit is until I read the book, *The Anatomy of Spirit* by Carolyn Myss. In her book, she out lined we have seven energy centers in our body, so called "Chakras," which are the language of our spirit and energy. Chakras are the centers of swirling energy, located along our spine from the base of the spine to the top of our head. Each chakra emits energy on specific energy wavelengths which influence the organs, muscles, ligaments and all other systems within its energy field. Chakras also influence the endocrine system and are strongly involved with our moods, personality and overall health.

Mona Lisa Schulz, M.D, PHD wrote a book *The Intuitive Advisor*. In her book, she described in detail how each chakra affects our health. If the chakras are connected and the flow of energy is smooth, we are healthy and full of energy. If the chakras are disconnected or blocked, we become emotionally ill and diseases may set in.

According to Dr. Schulz, the seven major chakras and associated diseases are:

1. Root chakra is the color red, located deep in the pelvis, slightly anterior to the rectum. This relates to our relationship with our tribes: family and society. When we grew up in an environment not loving or abusive, the root chakra is blocked. We feel insecure and it goes into a survival mode whenever we perceive there is danger. Many diseases are associated with this chakra, such as chronic fatigue syndrome, bone and joint issues and autoimmune diseases.

2. Womb chakra is the color orange, located at lower abdomen where the ovaries and the uterus lie. This second chakra is associated with creativity and the balance of relationships between money and love. Diseases that are associated with this chakra include low back pain, urinary tract infection, PMS, fibroid and infertility.

3. Solar plexus is the color yellow, located at stomach area, this represents our relationship with our self; the self-esteem. We have to build strong self-esteem and balance it with responsibilities otherwise we can develop diseases in the digestive tract, such as reflux, eating disorders, obesity or addictions.

4. Heart chakra is the color green, located at the middle of our body at the heart level. This relates to our basic emotions such as fear, anger, sadness, love or joy. We have to balance these emotions with our partnerships. Diseases associated with this chakra are heart attack, hypertension, palpitation, panic attack, asthma, emphysema, or breast cancer.

5. Throat chakra is the color light blue and is located at the mid neck/ throat area. This represents our power of will and communication. When our throat chakra is blocked, we are not able to express ourselves or stand up for ourselves. Thyroid diseases, throat or mouth diseases are associated with this chakra.

6.   Third eye chakra is the color purple and is located on our forehead just above and between our eyes. This chakra involves the power of our mind. Diseases of the brain or mental illness are related to this chakra.

7.   Crown chakra is the color white and is located at the top of head. This is our spiritual connection to the divine; our spirituality. When this chakra is out of balance we lose the purpose of life, serious illnesses can happen which may lead to death.

Most people's ailments are rooted to the imbalance of the first three chakras and/or the chakras being disconnected. How do we improve our chakras energy and balance? There are energy exercises and chakra meditations we can do to improve the energy flow. I recommend *Mind Mastery Meditation* by Valerie Hunt, and *Energy Medicine* by Donna Eden. There are other ways to improve our energy and vibration, such as doing the things you enjoy and by exercising in nature and absorbing the nature's energy. Yoga and Qi Gong are also ancient methods frequently used to help regain our energy.

However, the most important way to improve our chakra health is through the sixth chakra which is the power of our mind. Our mind chakra creates thoughts and emotions which influence all the other chakras.

In the book by Candice Pert, PhD *The Molecules of Emotion*, she points out that our emotions may trigger the secretion of neuropeptide which stimulates the receptors present on most of our body's cells. So the mind is not just in our brain but is distributed all over our body. In the book *Biology of Belief*, Bruce Lipton states that the mind (energy) and body (matter) are entangled. However positive thoughts alone are not enough to change our body, it also requires our subconscious mind to believe it is true for it to happen. Placebo effect has been well known over the years in the medical community, which is the due to the power of positive belief. Nocebos, the power of negative belief, is equally as effective in damaging our health!

Training for Positive Thoughts and Emotions

Now that we know how important our mind and emotion is to our health, how do we train our mind and emotion to be positive? How do we achieve long lasting peace and happiness? Here are some principles:

- Happiness is a state of mind that can be trained and cultivated. You do not have to be wealthy or famous to be happy. Happiness is a choice and a decision.

In *The Art of Happiness*, author Howard Cutler, M.D., has a conversation with the Dalai Lama, who says that the first step in seeking happiness is learning. Learn that negative emotions such as anger and hatred are not only bad and harmful to you personally but harmful to society and the future of the whole world. Once we realize that, we become determined to develop and cultivate positive emotions such as kindness, compassion and love.

To cultivate positive emotions, you first need to reduce negative emotions. Your thoughts impact your emotions. Indeed, negative thoughts foster negative emotions. It is very important, therefore, to think positively. You can see your glass as half full or half empty. That depends on what you perceive and your attitude in response to your perception. Try to find the good in everything and each person. Try to catch yourself before you fall into the negative thoughts and emotions that drag you down or sabotage you.

Changing our thoughts begins with being aware of our thoughts and consciously changing them when needed. I recommend the book *Ask and it's Given the Teaching of Abraham*, by Ester and Jerry Hicks. It teaches you how to improve your emotions by actively changing your thoughts thus improving your vibrational energy. We are all humans and experience human difficulties and emotions. Only those that train their mind to turn negative thoughts into positive thoughts and emotions through difficult challenges will be rewarded with happiness and good health. All of us can do this if we consciously work at it.

Our Belief System — Philosophy Toward Life

Our belief and value system is like the compass that guides our thoughts and decisions. It is better to have a belief system that is in line with our higher source so it's easier to achieve our emotional well-being. Here are a few principles:

- View difficulties as opportunities to grow.

  o   If we can develop an attitude that things happen for a reason, and bad things may just be a blessing in disguise. If we can train our mind to focus on the solution of the problem and not dwell on the negative emotions associated with it, we will handle difficulties in life much easier. It is helpful to remember that we are never alone in our suffering. Staying close to those in our support system at such a time can be quite sustaining when difficulties arise.

- Living in the present.

  o   Often we can be so caught up in our daily life that we miss out on pleasurable moments.

  o   Yesterday is history, tomorrow is mystery, and we only have today, the present. If we live in regret we live in the past. If we worry a lot we live thinking that in the future something bad will happen. We need to learn from our mistakes made in the past and to plan for the future, but we only have today for actually living. If we enjoy this moment, we can make today a better yesterday; that is the beginning of real effectiveness. If we do not live in the now, in our present moment, we are not truly living and savoring our lives!

- Detachment

  o   According to Buddhism, attachment is an illusion that causes suffering, while detachment leads you out of suffering. We think we own our life, our children, our spouse, our house, our health and wealth. In reality, this is an illusion and you can lose any of them at any time.

  o   When we see through the illusion and let go of the attachment, we will be able to appreciate and enjoy what is loaned to us and achieve long lasting peace and happiness.

- Cause and Effect
  - o We do not often stop to think about how our actions affect our well-being. But it is a fact that for every choice we make and each action we take, there is a consequence.
  - o For every unpleasant thing we are experiencing we are a part of the cause. Don't blame others for your misery. Examine why you are not taking actions to decrease the quotient of displeasure. The results you see today are from the causes you did or did not plan in the past. If you plan the cause today, you will see the result in the future. Take responsibility for your life; and remember you are the creator of your own life.
- Forgiveness toward Ourselves and Others
  - o Humans make mistakes, sometimes on purpose and oftentimes by accident. When a mistake occurs, the damage done can be physical or emotional, or both. In fact, words can do more damage than knives sometimes, so choose your words wisely.
  - o It is important to forgive ourselves and others. When you cannot find it within you to forgive yourself, you will ultimately feel guilty and depressed. The healthier approach is to view the mistake you have made as an opportunity to learn and to try not to repeat the same mistake. Apologize sincerely if you have hurt another. Try to make it up to the other party. If we do not forgive others, we continue to fill ourselves with anger, hatred, and resentment. These negative emotions will destroy our happiness, so we will ultimately pay the price for the mistakes made by others. Only through forgiveness can we let go of the pain. Then we can move on and heal our wounds.
- Acceptance and letting go
  - o We often prefer to look the other way when we cannot release something that no longer serves us well. Our rigid patterns can be a major source of

our suffering and sorrow. Then there are times when things just do not seem to go our way. We have been diligent and worked hard for important goals, but we may be thwarted by seemingly insurmountable obstacles. Or perhaps someone else is a source of profound difficulty, and nothing we do helps to improve that troubled relationship.

- o Knowing how to change circumstances is difficult at best. This is when the principle of acceptance comes into play. Do your best and let go, you may find the solution unfold in its own way.

- Love, gratitude, joy and peace
    - o Love is the highest form of energy. Love is seeing what other people need before they even think to ask for help. Love is kind words and constructive suggestions, not criticism. We do need to love ourselves first before we can give love to other people. Being appreciative and showing gratitude for simple things will bring tremendous joy and happiness in our life. Knowing all is well, will bring us peace. Positive emotions will increase your energy and sense of well-being.

- Purpose of Life
    - o Purpose of life is what keeps us going no matter what difficulties we are experiencing. Purpose of life is what makes life worthwhile living. Purpose of life brings the joy and sense of achievement in life. Purpose of our life is related to the crown chakra. People living without purpose are people that have lost their souls, and they are the saddest people.

We are all precious and holy children of God. We all have different talents that God has given us. We just need to find them and use them over the course of our lives. This will make us passionate, creative, happy, and productive. If we are happy, we can spread the happiness to other people. Living in such a way carries within itself the seeds of soul satisfaction and self-respect. Don't let the false purpose such as money, sex or power deter you from the true happiness.

Our spirit is a part of our daily existence; it is between our body and our mind. It is emotional energy that we can work on and improve. We are all on different levels of spiritual pathways. Let's help each other to reach higher levels so the world can be a better place!

Part IV: Healthy Aging Program

Chapter 15

Prevention of Disease

Reaching mid-life can be a wonderful time in our lives, one filled with happiness, prosperity, and a deep sense of fulfillment. Thanks to integrated approaches like pellet therapy that help us to balance the vital aspects of our health needs, we know that reaching middle-age does not have to herald a decline in our health and well-being. Physically, we can be as vital as ever, affording the time and energy we need to look back, treasure the lessons we have learned and share our experiences with others in anticipation of many happy and vital years to come.

While it is true that mid-life is a time when our bodies become more susceptible to chronic and debilitating diseases, there are a remarkable number of preventative measures you can take to dramatically improve and maintain your health, as well as forestall most debilitating diseases. The key to prevention is awareness. This chapter examines some of the most pressing diseases that pose particular risks to those in the mid-life stage, as well as discusses steps that can be taken to strengthen the body's internal systems, stay healthy, and prevent the onset of disease.

Cardiovascular Disease — Hypertension, Heart Attack, and Stroke

Cardiovascular disease affects heart and blood vessels. It is the number one killer of men and women worldwide. In the United States alone, it accounts for over 40 percent of all deaths, more than all forms of cancer combined.

Heart disease develops gradually over many years due to atherosclerosis, or hardening of the arteries. Healthy arteries are strong and flexible. As the walls of the arteries become thick and stiff, blood circulation is reduced. When an artery becomes totally occluded (blocked), the surrounding tissues are then blocked from their supply of oxygen and nutrients delivered by the blood vessels. As a result, the surrounding tissues die, which triggers a heart attack if the tissue is in the heart, or a stroke if the tissue is in the brain.

For many years, cholesterol has been singled out as a major culprit of hardening of the blood vessels. More and more recent evidence, however, shows that inflammation of the blood vessels also plays an important role in the cause of atherosclerosis.

A common illustration explains this point. If you cook food in a new pan with a nonstick surface, the food will not adhere to the pan. When the pan has been used frequently food begins to stick to the surface where it has been scratched. The same principle applies to blood vessels.

Blood vessels are very smooth, and normally cholesterol will not deposit in the arterial walls. When the blood vessels become inflamed, their surface becomes roughened. This allows cholesterol, along with calcium and other materials, to attach to the arterial wall resulting in the formation of plaque. As the plaque grows on the lining of the blood vessel wall, the wall itself can rupture, leading to occlusion of the artery, causing the occurrence of a heart attack or stroke. Or, circulation can get sluggish enough that the blood cells and platelets clump together and form a clot that blocks the blood vessel.

This, too, results in either a heart attack or stroke. It also explains why many people can have a heart attack or stroke while still showing normal levels of cholesterol. The heart attack or stroke is due to the underlying inflammation of the blood vessel wall that precipitates the formation of plaque. This is why normalizing the cholesterol level does not completely prevent cardiovascular disease.

What causes inflammation of the blood vessels? While there is much about inflammation that is not yet known, the causes for inflammation in the blood vessels that we do know about are free radicals, oxidative stress from lack of antioxidants due to inadequate nutrition, or exposure to environmental hazards such as smoking, toxins and heavy metals. Inflammation is a condition to be avoided as much as possible, as it also is a significant causative factor of cancer, arthritis, autoimmune diseases, Alzheimer's disease and premature aging as well as many other diseases.

We know inflammation devours nitric oxide, which leads to constriction of the blood vessels. Stress hormones, such as epinephrine (adrenaline) and norepinephrine, also constrict blood vessels. Constriction of blood vessel walls leads to an increase in blood pressure; the increased pressure on the blood vessels also contributes to inflammation. It becomes a vicious cycle. This is the physiology of how long-term stress, environmental toxins, and nutritional deficiency, along with other factors such as lack of exercise, obesity, smoking, and diabetes lead to hypertension and cardiovascular disease.

Diagnostic Tests for Screening Cardiovascular Diseases

1. Lipid panel
   a. The lipid panel includes triglycerides, high-density lipoproteins (HDL, or good cholesterol), and low-density lipoproteins (LDL, or bad cholesterol), total cholesterol, and HDL/LDL ratio. More advanced testing will include small, dense LDL; and Lp(a) (very dense LDL). Both are smaller than the larger buoyant LDL and can enter blood vessels easier, and cause atherosclerosis.

2. CRP (C-reactive protein)
   a. CRP (C-reactive protein) is an inflammation indicator. Hs-CRP (highly sensitive CRP) is a more specific indicator for blood vessel inflammation.[69,70]

3. Homocysteine
   a. Many studies link an increased homocysteine level with the risk of heart attack and stroke.[71] Homocysteine damages the blood vessel wall and leads to inflammation. Elevated homocysteine is

usually due to inadequate detoxification. It can be reduced in two ways. The first is methylation, a major process in phase II liver detoxification pathway. This occurs when methyl groups are assimilated by homocysteine and it becomes methionine (an amino acid), and S-adenosyl methionine (SAMe). This process requires the vitamin folic acid and vitamin B12. The second is a process called trans-sulfuration, where homocysteine is converted to cysteine.

b. This process requires vitamin B6. I interpret a higher homocysteine level as meaning that the body needs more help in the detoxifying process. A normal homocysteine level is below 15 μmol/L, while an optimal level is under 7 μmol/L. Take vitamins B6, B12 and folic acid, if your homocysteine level is not in the optimal range.

4. Fibrinogen

a. Fibrinogen is a protein involved in the formation of blood clots. A higher fibrinogen level leads to increased platelet aggregation and hyper-coagulation. This can be dangerous, especially if the blood vessel linings are inflamed. The inflammation attracts platelets and fibrinogen to form blood clots that block the arteries, often with disastrous results. Many people take a blood thinner such as aspirin to prevent the platelet aggregation that leads to heart attacks and strokes. Natural sources for platelet aggregation inhibitors are vitamin E, green tea, garlic, and ginkgo biloba.

5. Insulin, Blood Sugar, and HbA1c

a. By illustration, when you make dough for home baked bread it is very soft, but becomes hard as it is baked. Just as baking bread hardens the soft dough, a higher blood sugar level creates changes in protein structures. Hemoglobin (Hb) is a protein that changes into HbA1c in proportion to higher blood sugar levels. Thus it is a standard test to screen for diabetes and to follow in patients with diabetes. The normal range for HbA1c is under 6 percent; below 5.2% is optimal. Higher sugar intake triggers increased insulin production from the pancreas to handle the elevated sugar load. The protein conversion and higher insulin level ultimately leads to atherosclerosis, heart attacks and strokes, which happens in many patients with diabetes.

6. Body Scan

    a. A body scan is a radiology test that screens for calcification of blood vessels in the body. It is not 100 percent accurate because if the plaque is not calcified it will not show up in the scan. However, it can screen for atherosclerosis at an early stage. Other tests, such as the treadmill, echocardiogram, or Cardiolite nuclear testing, are not able to pick up early stages of atherosclerosis.

Prevention of Cardiovascular Disease

There are many proactive steps you can take today to reduce your risk of cardiovascular disease.

1. Diet

    a. Eating a nutritious and balanced diet that is high in fruits and vegetables helps to reduce inflammation, cholesterol, and homocysteine. For details see the anti-inflammation diet in chapter 9.

2. Exercise

    a. Regular exercise is essential to good health. It helps reduce blood pressure by dilating blood vessels, increasing endorphins; improving muscle tone; strengthening the heart, lungs and bones; lowering cholesterol; and reducing weight. Furthermore, exercise helps the body to detoxify by improving blood circulation and lymphatic drainage. Vigorous exercise also stimulates the secretion of growth hormone, which has many beneficial effects upon the body. Yoga and Qigong are relaxing exercises that can help to effectively reduce blood pressure.

3.   Stress Reduction

   a.   Positive thinking, meditating, deep breathing, getting adequate sleep, managing time wisely, building good relationships, controlling anger, and finding a purpose for your life are all important to reduce stress, and to better adjust to stressful situations. This also helps to keep your hormones and body chemicals in proper balance.

Balance Your Hormones

Testosterone for men and estrogen for women are known to improve cardiovascular health. High cortisol, adrenaline, and high insulin levels lead to high blood pressure and inflammation of blood vessel walls. Check your hormone levels and treat hormone deficiency adequately.

1.   Supplements

   a.   Recommended daily doses of supplements include:

      i.   Chelated magnesium 400-800 mg; and potassium, 500-800 mg, which may help blood vessel dilation and reduce blood pressure.[72]

      ii.   Co-Q10, 100-300 mg; and L-carnitine, 100-200 mg, which may improve mitochondria energy production and heart function.

      iii.   Arginine, 3,000 mg, stimulates the production of the potent vasodilator nitrous oxide as well as the secretion of growth hormone.

      iv.   Folic acid (folate), 800 mcg; vitamin B6, 100 mg; and vitamin B12, 400 mcg, which help to lower homocysteine and assist in the detoxification process.

      v.   Vitamin C, 1,000 mg; vitamin E, 400-800 IU; selenium, 100 mg; and beta-carotene,

vi.   25,000 IU, which are all antioxidants that neutralize free radicals.

vi.   Omega-3 fatty acids, 1,500 mg, are important in reducing inflammation of the blood vessels.

vii.   Fiber, such as grounded flaxseed fiber 1-2 tablespoons with each meal helps to reduce fat and sugar absorption. It also helps with cholesterol excretion.

Cancer

The big "C" is a terrifying word. It is the second most common cause of death in all age groups, but it is the number one cause of death in people under seventy years old.

The most common cancers are of the lung, colon, breast and prostate. In 1970 President Nixon declared war on cancer, expecting to find a cure by 1990. Unfortunately, the rate of cancer has increased instead, especially the hormone-dependent cancers such as breast and prostate cancer.

Cancer is often due, among other factors, to DNA mutation. What causes this mutation? Inflammation, particularly resulting from exposure to environmental toxins can lead to the development of cancer.[73,74] I believe cancer is mostly due to environmental factors, such as chronic stress, smoking and toxin exposure, but genetic predisposition also plays a significant role, probably through inadequate detoxification enzymes.

Diagnostic Testing for Early Cancer Detection

There are several approaches to screening for cancer; including history and physical exam, blood tests, radiological tests, and additional tests.

History and Physical Exam

Physicians will take a medical history of the patient and conduct a physical exam, which includes:

- Examining the thyroid nodule and lymph nodes.
- A digital rectal exam for rectal and prostate cancer.
- Breast palpation for unusual lumps.
- A skin inspection for pigmented lesions, moles or ulcerations that do not heal
- Blood Tests
  o The only blood test that is good for cancer screening is the PSA (prostate specific antigen) for prostate cancer. It is recommended once a year for men over fifty years old.
  o CEA for colon cancer and CA 125 for ovarian cancer, but these are not good for screening, primarily because these indicators do not show up until the later stages of cancer. Also, these indicators can increase due to benign conditions making them nonspecific which creates the need to rule out other causes. The best use of these two tests is to monitor for recurrence of cancer after treatment.
- Radiological Tests
  o There are several radiological tests that can be utilized to help detect certain forms of cancer.
    ▪ Mammograms. The mammogram for breast cancer screening is still standard and recommended by American Cancer Society to be done once a year for women over fifty years old. Unfortunately, the mammogram is not accurate when breast tissues are dense, thus it is not a good screening tool for women younger than 40 years old. The newer digital mammogram is better in terms of clarity.
    ▪ The breast MRI (magnetic resonance imaging) is also available now, but its use is limited due to cost. A breast ultrasound is usually done after the mammogram if there is an area with increased density. If questions persist, then the MRI is used for greater diagnostic resolution.

- Thermogram of the breast, which uses infrared imaging, has been around for a while but is not considered standard screening. The theory behind thermography is that if cancer cells are growing in a certain area, the blood supply and temperature of that location will increase. This makes it good for early detection, but it can be nonspecific due to other conditions, such as infection.

- Most importantly, women of all ages should learn how to do breast exams and do them regularly. I have seen patients who had a negative mammogram but had a palpable lump that a biopsy identified as cancer. If there is a strong family history of breast cancer, genetic testing for BRCA 1 and BRCA 2 may be valuable, too.

- Chest X-ray. A chest X-ray for lung cancer screening is recommended once a year for those over fifty years old, as well as for high-risk groups, chiefly smokers. CT (computer tomography) of the chest is more accurate, but its use is limited due to cost and radiation exposure. It is often used if the screening chest X-ray shows an abnormality suspicion for cancer.

- Colonoscopy. A lower GI (barium enema) or colonoscopy is done to screen for colon cancer. The preparation for both procedures is the same. The colonoscopy is more expensive and more invasive. It is recommended for high-risk populations, such as those with a family history of colon cancer, chronic inflammation of the bowel such as ulcerative colitis, Crohn's disease, irritable bowel syndrome, or chronic constipation. Generally, it is done once every ten years for people over fifty years old. This is frequent enough, unless a polyp (growth) is discovered; then a colonoscopy needs to be done every three to five years, with biopsies of any polyps for possible cancer.

- Endoscope. Endoscope is routinely performed in Japan as a screening test for stomach cancer because the Japanese have a high rate of stomach cancer. It is not routinely done in the U.S., but it is probably a good idea for people who have stomach problems, especially among the Asian population. Another very common cancer among Asians is liver cancer associated with chronic hepatitis B. For Asians an abdominal ultrasound is recommended yearly.

- Body scan. A body scan is a better tool for early detection of cancer and heart diseases. However, it is not 100 percent accurate and can have many false positives, which can lead to unnecessary procedures having to be performed. For those over fifty years old, I recommend that it be done every ten years.

Other Tests

Additional tests include Pap cytology for cervical cancer, and urinalysis for blood in the urine, which can be due to kidney or bladder cancer. Sputum cytology for lung cancer, if there is chronic productive cough, stool guaiac occult blood for colon cancer and biopsies for suspicious lumps or skin lesions that do not heal.

Cancer Prevention

There are many simple, yet powerful steps you can take to minimize your risk of cancer.

1. Avoid Cancer-causing (Carcinogenic) Sources
   a. Do not smoke, and avoid secondhand smoke.
   b. Avoid xenohormones or hormone disruptors, such as meat from animals raised with hormones, as well as pesticides, bug killers, and plastics.

c. Avoid processed foods that contain artificial food colors, sweeteners and preservatives.

d. Avoid hair dyes, cosmetics, perfumes or deodorants that contain toxic chemicals.

e. Avoid drinking chlorinated tap water.

f. Avoid wrapping food in plastic wrap or aluminum foil. Try to use glass containers.

2. Diet

a. A cancer-avoidance diet should focus on toxin avoidance and detoxification and include:

   i. Large numbers of servings of organically grown vegetables, especially cruciferous ones such as broccoli, cabbage, Brussels sprouts, and cauliflower, which help the liver detoxify and provide antioxidants to neutralize free radicals.

   ii. Citrus fruits; such as oranges, lemons, limes and tangerines that are high in vitamin C.

   iii. Increase fiber through vegetables or foods with ground flax seed.

   iv. Drink plenty of water: 50 percent of your weight in ounces (for example, 100 lbs. = 50 ounces).

   v. Reduce animal meats, especially those that are nitrate-cured or smoked, and high in animal fats.

   vi. Reducing sugar and other refined carbohydrates.

3. Stress Reduction

a. Be in tune with your inner child. Write down your feelings and emotions on a daily basis. Let go of the negative emotions, and cultivate the positive emotions.

b. Practice meditation, deep breathing and creative imaging. Regularly engage in relaxation exercises such as yoga.

    c.   Find a purpose in your life. Set goals. Plan for the future, and prioritize your activities.

    d.   Do simple things that bring you joy, such as walking on the beach, taking a relaxing bath, getting a massage, listening to your favorite music, or dancing. Do these activities regularly.

    e.   Associate frequently with good friends who are supportive, and do fun things together.

    f.   Laugh a lot. Laughter is the best medicine.

4.   Regular Exercise

    a.   Exercise has many overall health benefits. For cancer prevention, it improves circulation and aids in the detoxification process. Exercise also improves immunity by bringing more nutrition and oxygen to organs and tissues.

5.   Hormone Balance

    a.   Many hormones, such as estrogen, progesterone, testosterone and melatonin help with sleep quality. This leads to improved immunity and an overall sense of well-being. When we are feeling good and energetic, we tend to take better care of ourselves and others, too.

6.   Supplements

    a.   Antioxidants daily dosage includes vitamin C, 1,000 mg; vitamin E, 400-800 IU; beta-carotene, 25,000 IU; and selenium, 100 mg; all of which neutralize free radicals and help the detoxification process.

    b.   Fiber, such as ground flax seed, psyllium, or apple pectin helps the detoxification process.

    c.   Omega-3 fatty acids, 1,500 mg to help reduce inflammation.

Metabolic Syndrome — Insulin Resistance, Obesity, and Diabetes

Metabolic syndrome entails a collection of negative health factors that lead to developing insulin resistance, fatty degeneration of the liver, heart disease, and type II diabetes. It is estimated that over fifty million people in America fit into the clinical profile of metabolic syndrome. Indeed, more than 20 million people are diagnosed with diabetes and among those, 90 percent have type II (adult onset) diabetes. The remaining 10 percent have type I (juvenile) diabetes.

In the year 2000, the U.S. spent roughly $2 billion on the treatment of diabetes. Obesity, often a factor in diabetes, reached epidemic levels by the year 2000 and most members of this group already have, or are on their way to developing metabolic syndrome, diabetes, and heart disease, unless they change their lifestyle and eating habits.

Metabolic syndrome is a constellation of obesity, elevated cholesterol and triglycerides, along with a high insulin level. Insulin is a hormone manufactured by specialized glands in the pancreas that facilitate the transportation of sugar from the bloodstream into the tissues and cells. This syndrome begins with overeating; particularly high glycemic index carbohydrates, such as breads, pastas, potatoes, rice, or desserts. In response to an inundation of these high glycemic foods, the body secretes insulin to handle the sugar load.

A higher sugar load translates to higher insulin demand. If the body does not burn off the sugar immediately, it stores it in a lighter form, which is fat. As a person continues to eat sugars (carbohydrates), the body gains fat. Initially the fat goes primarily to the abdominal area, then the subcutaneous (under the skin) fat layers throughout the body, then the muscle, the whole body, and eventually to the liver. When this occurs, the condition is referred to as fatty liver.

Another factor in metabolic syndrome is insulin resistance.[75] As greater amounts of fat are stored in the cell membrane (outer covering), it becomes insensitive to insulin and the body has to secrete higher levels of insulin to handle the same sugar load. If a person continues to overeat foods loaded with high glycemic carbohydrates, even with increased production of insulin, the body cannot handle the sugar load. The result is the beginning of an increase in the blood sugar in the blood stream, which is type II diabetes.

Type I diabetes results from the pancreas being destroyed by a viral infection, or an autoimmune disease, which leads to its inability to secrete insulin. This form of diabetes usually starts at a much younger age and requires treatment by insulin injections. The treatment for type II diabetes is not insulin; it is simply life style change and supplements as we are going to discuss nest in more detail.

High insulin provokes inflammation by triggering pro-inflammatory cytokines. High insulin causes a lipoprotein lipase deficiency, which leads to increased triglycerides and decreased HDL (the good cholesterol). A fatty liver also contributes to increased inflammation, since the burdened liver is not able to detoxify as well as a normal liver. Toxins can certainly cause more inflammation. Inflammation of the blood vessel walls and high cholesterol leads to atherosclerosis (hardening of the arteries) and hypertension. Hypertension, diabetes and hyperlipidemia (high cholesterol) lead to heart attacks and strokes.

Laboratory Testing

When checking for diabetes and metabolic syndrome, these are the most common tests physicians will perform.

1. Insulin Level

    a. A normal fasting insulin level is 3 to 28; the optimal range is below 5.

2. HbA1c

    a. HbA1c is the most important test for diabetes. As stated earlier in this chapter, the normal range for HbA1c is 4.8% to 6.0%; below 5.2% is optimal, and should be measured every three months for diabetic patients.

3. Lipid Profile

Prevention and Treatment of Metabolic Syndrome

There are many things you can do to prevent and treat metabolic syndrome, starting with a diet to lose weight.

1. Weight loss diet. Please see Chapter 9 for detail information.

2. Supplements. It is very important to take supplements if you have metabolic syndrome in order to reduce inflammation, improve insulin sensitivity, lower cholesterol, and improve detoxification.

   a. Fiber slows down the absorption of glucose, increases the excretion of cholesterol, decreases constipation, and provides a feeling of fullness, which helps to reduce the appetite and thereby lose weight. However, water soluble fiber is fermented by intestinal bacteria and can cause gas, so it is better to start slowly. Fiber also needs to be taken with plenty of water. I recommend psyllium, ground flax seed, or natural fiber from fruits and vegetables. Take 1 tablespoon of fiber in a large glass of water or tea and drink it before or with meals.

   b. High-potency multiple vitamins and minerals provide a base of antioxidants and important vitamins and minerals, such as chromium, magnesium, vanadium, zinc, selenium, vitamins C, E, and B complex. These neutralize free radicals and promote better function of insulin.

   c. Omega-3 fish oil reduces inflammation. Use pharmaceutical grade to avoid heavy metals and environmental toxins.

   d. Herbs that can improve insulin functions and sensitivities such as gymnema sylvestre, American and Korean ginseng, and fenugreek.

   e. Coenzyme Q10, L-carnitine, and alpha lipoic acid, which helps with energy production and weight loss.

3. Exercise is absolutely an essential part of recovery from metabolic syndrome. Exercise directly improves insulin sensitivity and blood sugar. Other benefits are that it increases muscle mass and helps to burn off fat; it lowers total cholesterol and raises HDL (the good cholesterol); it burns off calories to help lose weight and it reduces blood pressure.

4. Stress reduction and lifestyle change. Do not smoke, as smoking generates a plethora of free radicals that damage the body. Do not drink alcohol, as it exacerbates a fatty liver. Stress increases cortisol, which leads to increased blood sugar and insulin. Stress also increases adrenaline, which elevates blood pressure.

5. Balance your hormones. Normal levels of testosterone and estrogen improve insulin sensitivity and function, which lead to healthy blood sugar levels. Adequate thyroid hormone levels are needed for energy production and weight loss. Get your hormones checked if you are overweight and have high blood pressure or high blood sugar.

6. Reduce exposure to environmental toxins and take detoxification supplements, since a fatty liver impairs the ability of the liver to detoxify properly.

7. An accumulation of toxins leads to more inflammation, sluggish metabolism and weight gain.

Premature Brain Aging, Memory Loss, Neurodegenerative Disease, Impaired

Cognition, and Dementia

Most parts of the body go through constant renewal. Skin cells regenerate each month, for instance, while red blood cells regenerate every four months. But we die with the same brain cells with which we were born. It is hard to regenerate brain cells. Once they are gone, they are usually gone forever.

Causes of Premature Brain Aging, dementia, and neurodegenerative diseases

It is frightening to think that the brain can die before the rest of the body, yet this is what occurs with dementia and other brain disorders. Here are contributors to this horrific condition:

- Chronic inflammation caused by toxins and free radicals.

- Nutritional deficiencies resulting from improper diet.

- Decreased oxygen and nutrients delivered to brain cells due to impaired circulation as a result of atherosclerosis, stroke or heart attack.

- Hormone deficiencies, especially testosterone, estrogen, and thyroid hormone.

- Poor lifestyle habits, such as smoking, excessive consumption of alcohol, street drugs, stress, and lack of exercise.

- Brain injuries due to trauma or accidents.

Prevention of Neurodegenerative Diseases

The consequences of brain cell loss can be catastrophic, but there are simple steps you can take right now to protect the health of your brain cells and minimize the risk of neurodegenerative diseases.

1. Commit to a healthy-aging diet geared toward reducing inflammation as outlined in chapter 9. Pay particular attention to:

    a. Ingest antioxidants from eating fresh organic fruits and vegetables.

    b. Avoid processed foods and bad fats.

    c. Foods rich in omega-3 fatty acids, especially DHA (docosahexaenoic acid), which is essential as the building blocks of the brain cell membranes.

    d. Eat good proteins as a source of amino acids that turn into neurotransmitters.

2. Avoid brain injuries. Wear protective headgear when riding a bike and participating in impact-sports.

3. Avoid using alcohol, tobacco or recreational drugs.

4. Avoid toxins as much as possible and detoxify as needed.

5. Make exercise a priority, especially aerobic exercise, which delivers more nutrients and oxygen to the brain cells. Exercise increases brain endorphins, nature's antidepressants. Deep breathing and relaxation exercises help relax the body and also increase the supply of oxygen to brain cells.

6. Exercise your brain.

   a. Learn new skills such as dancing or playing the piano.

   b. Engage in creative writing.

   c. Play chess or solve puzzles.

   d. Use your senses (touch, smell, vision and hearing) to stimulate brain functions by engaging in aromatherapy, music therapy, sculpture, or reading.

   e. Engage in social interactions. Meaningful conversation can improve thought processes.

7. Stress reduction.

   a. Positive thoughts, joyful moments, and laughter help the neuroendocrine system to work optimally.

8. Prevent diseases such as obesity, hypertension, cardiovascular disease and diabetes, which decrease the blood supply to the brain and impair its function.

9. Balance hormones. Replace hormone deficiencies; especially testosterone, estrogen, thyroid, melatonin, DHEA, and growth hormone.

10. Use nutritional supplements.

   a. Omega-3 fatty acids in fish oil. Fish has long been referred to as brain food because the basic building blocks of brain cell membrane are EPA (eicosapentaenoic acid) and DHA (docosahexaenoic acid), which are both derived from fish oil. These fatty acids also reduce inflammation, and thus help prevent premature brain aging.

b.   High potency antioxidants and minerals.

c.   Co-Q10, alpha lipoic acid and acetyl-L carnitine. All of these nutrients are needed in the mitochondria, which are the energy furnaces of the cell. Co-Q10, a coenzyme, is in all of the body's cells, particularly the heart and brain cells. These supplements help prevent brain aging by several different mechanisms, such as reducing free radicals and enhancing cellular energy and functions.

d.   Choline, an essential nutrient usually grouped with the vitamin B complex, and lecithin are the precursors to acetylcholine, the neurotransmitter involved in memory.

e.   Phosphatidylserine (PS) plays an important role in maintaining the brain cell membrane. By protecting the brain cell membrane, PS facilitates the transportation of nutrients into brain cells.

f.   Herbs such as ginkgo biloba and vinpocetine improve circulation to the brain.

Osteoporosis and Osteopenia

Osteoporosis is a systemic skeletal disease characterized by low bone mass which leads to increasing bone fragility and susceptibility to fracture. It is a very common diagnosis among older women and also happens in older men. Many women are put on prescription medication for this diagnosis which may cause fear and worry.

How is osteoporosis diagnosed since it does not have any symptoms? Usually, by bone density test such as DEXA (Duel-energy X ray absorptiometry). It concentrate X-ray in certain area of the body and measure the proportion of the light that pass through that tissue as an indicator of not being blocked by minerals in the bone. The computer then divided the number that represent the amount of light filtering through by the surface area of the bone being measured, thus come up with the Bone Mineral Density (BMD).

The standard peak bone density was set by a selected group of young adults, typically in their twenties, so called T score. If you match with 50 percentile of the young adult, your T score is 0. If you fall below negative 1.0 to 2.4 standard deviation, you have osteopenia. If you fall below -2.5 of the standard deviation, you have osteoporosis. However this test is not that accurate, due to the variation of bone density in different ethnic group, or you have small bone structure to begin with, or the machine use different technology.

Our bones are complex and dynamic living tissue and goes through constant remodeling. Bones are made of 65 percent mineralized collagen that gives the outer bone structure and 35 percent collagen matrix looks beehive as the inner bone structure. The collagen matrix is made of nutrients and minerals that give flexibility to the bone, also makes the bone more resistant to breaking. In the remodeling process, the old bone needs to be removed first by osteoclast, and new bone being formed by osteoblast. As we get older, less new bone is being formed due to the decline of the hormones yet the old bone is still being removed, thus cause thinning of the bone. This decline of bone formation happens significantly within five years of reaching menopause as the hormone levels decline dramatically.

How do we treat and prevent osteoporosis? Orthodox approach is using medication such as Boniva or Fosmax which works by blocking the bone absorption without helping new bone formation. They do increase bone density but does not reduce fracture. Picture a young tree branch, which is more flexible than an old dried up wood. If you keep the bone thicker but less flexible due to lack of new bones, it is not going to prevent fracture.

What is the real effective treatment of osteoporosis and osteopenia? Number one is hormone replacement treatment with the safest form bio-identical hormone pellet treatment.

There are other important treatments listed below:

1.   Alkaline diet

     a.   Our body is in mild alkaline state and if we change the pH just a little, it has tremendous influence on our body's chemical reactions. This is why our body tries it's best to maintain a constant pH level. Usually the kidneys are the major regulating organ by excrete acidity in the urine. However, as we grow older the kidneys may not work as efficiently, and our body compensates by pulling calcium out of the bone to reduce the acidity in our body. To prevent the calcium coming out from our bone, we need to avoid acidic foods and eat more foods that are alkaline producing. Most processed foods and meats are acidic, while most vegetables and fruits are alkaline. Drinking alkaline water can help too.

2. Supplement:

   a. Vitamin D and calcium come to mind but there are many minerals needed in the bones, such as magnesium, zinc, boron, manganese and silicon. Antioxidants such as Vitamin A, B, C, E and bioflavonoids reduce free radicals and promote cell growth such as osteoblast, the bone building cell. Taking a high potency high quality multiple vitamins with minerals is so important in slowing down aging and promote bone health.

3. Exercise:

   a. Weight bearing exercises such as walking or jogging are very important for bone growth because they make you move against the gravity in upright position. The bone cells can sense the mechanical changes in the environment, thus stimulate the bone growth. Another very important exercise is weight training to build muscles. Strong muscles stabilize the joints and prevent falls.

In today's world, people are living healthier and longer lives than ever before. As we age, it becomes much more essential to keep our body and mind fit in order to experience optimal energy, clarity, and balance in our day-to-day lives. Although reaching the mid-life stage can make us more susceptible to debilitating diseases, it is important to remember that taking simple steps to improve our well-being each day can make us stronger, healthier and far more resistant to aging and diseases than ever before.

Following the steps outlined in this chapter will go a long way towards improving and preserving your life-long health.

Chapter 16

8 Weeks to Vitality

Do you want to experience more energy each day? Do you want a clear, focused mind; an even, balanced mood; and a zest for life you have not known in years? It is within your reach. One of the most common questions I get from my patients is how to integrate all of the information I give them on improving their health into a workable, sustainable and successful program that meets their individual needs. In this chapter we are going to bring this experience to you by reviewing the entire program I use in my practice to help people achieve peak health and vitality.

Week 1 — Health Assessment

1. Questionnaire for Health Assessment
Answer each question based on the following symptoms:
Point scale:
0 = never or almost never happens
1 = occasionally happens, the degree is not severe
2 = occasionally happens, the degree is severe
3 = frequently happens, the degree is not severe
4 = frequently happens, the degree is severe

Head
    Headache
    Dizziness
Eyes
    Watery
    Itching

Blurred vision
Ears
Ringing in ears
Hearing loss
Earache or infection
Nose
Sneezing
Congestion
Postnasal drip
Mouth
Sore throat
Hoarseness
Gum infection
Toothache
Canker sores
Discolored tongue
Skin and Hair
Acne
Hives
Rash
Dry skin
Hair loss
Hot flashes
Heart
Palpitations or irregular heartbeat
Chest pain
Shortness of breath on exertion
Leg edema (swelling) Lungs
Cough
Asthma attack
Shortness of breath
Digestive tract
Nausea/vomiting
Diarrhea
Constipation
Bloating or gas
Heartburn
Abdominal pain
Joints/Muscles

Joint pain or stiffness
Muscle pain/body ache
Neck pain
Back pain

Weight
Weight gain
Weight loss
Craving certain foods
Binge eating/drinking
Difficulty losing weight

Energy
Easily fatigued
Difficulty getting up
Lethargy, difficulty functioning
Cold intolerance
Cold hands and feet
Restless/hyperactive

Sleep
Difficulty falling asleep
Restless sleep
Frequent nightmares
Wake up frequently
Sleep too much

Emotions
Mood swings, moodiness
Anxiety, nervousness
Anger/irritability
Depression/loss of interest

Brain
Poor memory
Mental fog
Difficulty concentrating
Difficulty learning
Confusion
Headache

Immune System
Frequent illness
Autoimmune disease
Allergies/hay fever

Gyn/Urinary tract
    Frequent urination
    Nocturia (excessive urination at night)
    Incontinence
    Urinary tract infection
    Genital itching or discharge
    Vaginal dryness or painful intercourse

Total Score

Results Analysis

If your score is under five, your general health is good. Between five and fifty, it is time to take a proactive stand toward making changes that will enhance your body's health. If you have a score above fifty, you are heading toward, or facing major medical issues. This also means that you need to seek medical evaluation and treatment.

    This self-assessment can also be repeated over time to determine if you are moving upward or downward. If the score is coming down, you are improving. If the score is increasing, you are edging closer to health problems.

Laboratory Assessment

One of the first steps in helping to determine your current state of health is to run some general and specific tests.

- General:
  - Blood tests, including CBC, liver and kidney functions, lipid panel, and urinalysis.
- Specific:
  - Fasting insulin, HbAlc: screen for diabetes and metabolic syndrome.
  - Homocysteine, fibrinogen, hs-CRP: screen for cardiovascular risk factors.
  - Hormone panels: screen for thyroid, adrenal and sex hormones.
  - Toxins and infections, such as heavy metals, H pylori or candida antibody

Week 2 — Hormone Balance

This week is the first consultation, physical examination and hormone evaluation treatment. Hormone balance starts with bio-identical hormone replacement for both men and women if the sex hormone levels are low. I also treat subclinical hypothyroidism during this visit. Adrenal function is assessed and treated as needed. The benefits of hormones that are balanced and at youthful levels are numerous, not the least of which is enhancing the quality of life of any individual at any age. It is also a necessary step to achieve vitality.

Week 3 — Make Sleep a Priority, Check Your Stress Inventory, and Take Control

Part I. Make Sleep a Priority

With the help of hormones, you should be sleeping better now. Here are other strategies to try if you still have trouble sleeping:

1. Minimize or Avoid Stimulants.
    a. Avoid alcohol.
    b. Avoid caffeine containing beverages or foods after 12 noon. This includes Pepsi, Coke, coffee or espresso, lattes, and chocolate.
    c. Avoid Sudafed or other over-the-counter decongestants.
    d. Avoid aerobic exercise after 6 P.M. Do relaxing exercise at night such as yoga or Pilates.

2. Avoid Nighttime Tension and Anxiety.
    a. Avoid watching violent or anxiety provoking news, TV programs or movies at night.
    b. Avoid paying bills or checking the stock market before bedtime.
    c. Avoid arguments at night. Schedule difficult conversations at a time during the day when both parties are not emotionally disturbed. Try to achieve

some resolution of the difficult issues if you have an argument before bedtime.

3.   Sleep Planning.

   a.   Plan to sleep eight to nine hours a day and keep it the same time every day to train your biological clock. Plan to go to bed before 11:00 p.m. If you can go to bed around 9:00 p.m. to 10:00 p.m., it is even better.

   b.   Avoid large meals or spicy food at least three hours before bed time.

   c.   Avoid drinking liquid at least two hours before bedtime. Make sure you empty your bladder before going to bed so that you do not have to get up at night to go to the bathroom.

4.   Bedroom Preparation

   a.   Keep your bedroom air clean, especially if you have nasal congestion or are prone to snoring. Use a HEPA air filter if needed. You can use the filter for four to six hours before bedtime if the noise bothers you.

   b.   Keep your bedroom quiet. Turn off any appliances or clocks that make noise.

   c.   Close the window or use ear plugs if necessary.

   d.   Decrease the light in your bedroom by turning the light off, using a window curtain, or wearing eye shades.

   e.   Make sure the bed, pillow, and mattress are comfortable.

   f.   Make sure the temperature in the bedroom is not too hot or too cold. Use appropriate bed covers.

   g.   Avoid sleeping near electric fields. Try to keep your head at least five feet away from electric fields generated by electrical outlets, radios, clocks, computers and night lights. Avoid using an electric blanket or water bed.

5. Strategies for Falling Asleep or Staying Sleep

   a. Daily journal your emotions and feelings. Be in touch with your inner child. If there are things that worry you, write them down. Ask yourself how likely this is going to happen, and if this is likely to happen, ask yourself what you can do to be prepared. If this very unlikely to happen, ask yourself if you can release the unnecessary worry or fear.

   b. Most thoughts are recurrent thoughts. Write them down so that you do not have to think it over and over again. Meditate afterward.

   c. Write down the things you need to do tomorrow and prioritize them.

   d. Relaxation exercise such as yoga, deep breathing, and creative visualization help to unwind your busy brain waves. Use a relaxation CD or soothing music or nature sounds.

   e. If you still have trouble with sleep due to unresolved emotional issues, consider counseling.

6. Supplements for Sleep

   a. Melatonin 0.5 mg to 2 mg sublingual before sleep.

   b. Magnesium 400 mg to 600 mg before bedtime helps to relax the muscles and allows you to sleep deeper.

   c. Amino acids such as tryptophan, 5-HTP, and SAMe help to increase serotonin and GABA.

   d. Herbs such as valerian root or passionflower help with relaxation and sleep.

Part II. Check Your Stress Inventories and Take Control

Scientists studying the events that cause the most mental and emotional stress discovered that they have four characteristics in common. We are stressed by:

1. Things that are new to us.

2. Unpredictability.

3. Sense of threat.
4. Loss of control.

Life events that cause most stressful responses:

1. Death of spouse or a close family member.
2. Law suit or detention in jail.
3. Marital separation or divorce.
4. Major personal injuries or illness.
5. Major change in financial state.
6. Loss of job or being fired.
7. Changing to a different line of work, or starting new school.
8. Foreclosure on a mortgage.
9. Conflict/tension with spouse, children, in laws or other family members.
10. Major change in living conditions (moving, remodeling, etc.).

Sources of Stress

1. Work

Are you overwhelmed?

- Reorganize your work surroundings for better efficiency.
- Use an organizer to plan your day and organize tasks by priority.
- Are you losing self-control or the ability to control normal events?
- Recognize the things that you can control and forget about controlling the rest.
- If you always feel the need to control others or life events you may want to consider professional counseling.

Do you have difficult co-workers?

- Resolve issues with supervisors and co-workers as soon as possible.
- Develop positive communication and interaction skills.

Do you hate your job?

- Find another job that you like.
- You may need more training or schooling. Make plans for a slow transition if there is financial difficulty.

2. Relationships

Relationships with our immediate family and our friends are like the fruit trees and flowers in the garden. If you planted them early and attended them regularly with love, they will bloom with beautiful flowers and yield delicious fruits. Great relationships yield great love, which is what sustains humankind. Many relationship problems are rooted in power struggles, self-centeredness, a lack of appreciation, and communication.

Write down a list of people you enjoy being with. Make calls or arrange visits regularly so you can find joy in friendship

Cultivate gratitude. Being thankful and expressing your appreciation to others is therapeutic. Many times we forget to do it with those people we see each day; our co-workers, our spouse, our children or our parents. Remind yourself to write down things and people you are thankful for and make a habit to express your gratitude.

Resolve your disputes. Relationships will eventually produce conflict. Some are minor and some are major. If left unresolved and the longer you wait, the minor ones will become major, and the major ones will become un-resolvable. Make a list of people you need to resolve disputes with, and try resolving the smallest one first then move on to the next. You will find you are much less stressed, and empowered, once you have solved those conflicts.

Forgiveness: There are times other people genuinely hurt us, physically or emotionally. Regardless of the offense, if we are unwilling to forgive, the bitterness, anger, and resentment in us will further hurt us and lead to more stress in our life. Make a list of persons you are unwilling to forgive and if you still cannot forgive them even though you tried, seek counseling with a therapist or a spiritual leader. There are times we hurt other person, consider asking forgiveness from that person and reconcile the relationship. We also need to forgive ourselves too, so the burden of guilt can be lifted.

3. Finances

Financial instability creates tremendous anxiety and stress. When an economic downturn strikes, everybody feels stressed. It is a good time to reassess our needs and wants. It is a good habit to live within our means. In the past many consumers over-extended their lifestyle; perhaps it is time to cut back and rearrange your priorities. Ask what we can learn from the situation. Remember, the most important things in life cannot be bought with money, and we do not need a lot of money to sustain our basic living.

- Downsize. Simplify your life.
- Create a plan to stabilize your financial situation.
- Recognize that it might take time, but with a good plan in place, you can stop worrying.

4. Health Issues

Many health issues can be improved by simple steps:

- Take actions to stop bad habits such as smoking or drinking alcoholic beverages.
- Implement good habits such as daily exercise, eating healthy meals, and taking supplements (this is your next week's home work).
- See a physician who can help you uncover any illness.

Week 4 — Better Nutrition and Healthy Diet

This week, start following the health aging diet that is in Chapter 9. Now is a good time to check your pantry. Throw out oils and seasonings that are over six months old. Get rid of cookies, candies, ice cream, cakes, diet soda, chips, and instant noodles, canned and processed foods. Buy organic virgin olive oil and cold pressed vegetable oils of your choice. Buy organic seasonings, sea salt, and raw organic nuts and seeds.

Plan your weekly meals ahead of time so that you do not have to eat on the run or eat junk fast food. Do not eat in a restaurant or eat fast food more than twice per week. You will save a lot of money this way, money that can be used to buy organic fruits, vegetables, nuts, and seeds. Make chicken soup or bake meats during the weekend so you can use them during the week. There are a lot of delicious recipes for soups, salads, and main dishes that you can find on the internet or get from your favorite cook books.

If you are still buying bottled water or drinking from the tap, install a reverse osmosis water filter under your kitchen sink so you can get clean and filtered water.

The principle of healthy diet is eating the foods our ancestors use to eat. That is, organic fruit, vegetables, nuts seeds and lean meat or seafood in its natural form. Avoid overeating. Avoid processed foods high in carbohydrates such as breads, pastas, cakes, and cookies. Also avoid processed meats, fish or cheese. Here are a few of my favorite recipes and all are less than 400 calories;

Smoothies:

I love smoothies for breakfast because they are delicious, nutritious, and easy to make. I also add medical food such as inflamCore or SP complete for additional nutritional value. The recipes below each makes 16 oz. smoothie:

Very Berry

1/3 cup blueberries, frozen or fresh
1/3 cup strawberries
1/3 cup raspberries
1 tsp. agave or dash of stevia
1 cup coconut milk

Immune Blast

1 banana
1 inch ginger
1/2 lemon, peeled

1/2 apple, cored
3-4 pitted dates
1 cup water

Green Lean

3/4 cup mango, frozen or fresh
1 cup orange juice
1/2 tsp. cinnamon
1 cup spinach or kale

Nuts Coco

1/2 soaked brazil nuts
1 banana
1tablespoon cacao powder
1teaspoon maca powder (optional)
1 cup fresh coconut meat or 1/2 cup dried coconut

Salads:

I eat a salad for lunch every day. I use seasonal vegetables such as lettuces, spinach, tomatoes, red or yellow pepper. I also use celery, dried or fresh fruits such as apple, grapes, strawberry, cranberry or raisin, with nuts, such as almond, walnut or cashew. I add avocado and olive oil for good fat, vinegar and salt for taste. It's simple yet delicious.

Asian Cucumber Sesame Salad

Ingredients:

1 large cucumber sliced
1 teaspoon sesame seed
2 tablespoons apple cider vinegar
1 table spoon fresh lemon juice
1 teaspoon sesame oil

Directions:

Mix ingredients together, marinate for 15 minutes or more, serve chilled.

Asparagus Apple Salad

Ingredients:

6-8 stalks of asparagus chopped
1 apple diced (or use strawberry instead)
4 Tablespoon lemon juice
1/4 teaspoon cinnamon
1 table spoon finely minced onion dash of sea salt and pepper
1 tablespoon olive oil or coconut oil

Directions:

Boil asparagus in water for 1 minute, toss with oil and lemon juice, apple, onion and spice.

Serve hot or cold.

Coleslaw

Ingredients

1/4 head red cabbage, shredded
1/4 head green shredded cabbage
1 carrot, shredded
1 apple diced (optional)

Dressing

2 tablespoon lemon juice
1 tablespoon apple cider vinegar
1 table spoon olive oil
A dash of cinnamon, sea salt and pepper stevia or agave to the taste
Toss all the ingredients together, allow to marinate overnight or serve immediately

Soups

Hot and sour Thai Shrimp Soup

Ingredients

100gm shrimp

2 cup vegetable broth
1/2 lemon juice with rind
1 lemon grass stalk
2-3 slice of fresh ginger
red pepper or cayenne pepper
1 tablespoon green onion
1 tablespoon fresh chopped cilantro dash of salt

Directions

Bring the broth to boil. Add ginger, lemongrass, lemon juice, onion and pepper. Simmer for ten minutes, add shrimp, cook for another five to eight minutes. Serve hot with cilantro on top.

Cream of asparagus soup,

Ingredients

1 tablespoon soaked raw cashews
1 tablespoon soaked raw Brazil nuts
1/2 cup water
1 tablespoon miso paste
1/2 pound fresh asparagus, chopped
1 garlic clove in hot water
cilantro for garnishing

Directions:

Place the cashews and Brazil nuts in water in a blender and blend until smooth. Add miso, asparagus, and garlic. Blend again. Add very hot water in 1 to 1 ratio before serving the soup. Garnish with cilantro. You can substitute broccoli or cauliflower for the asparagus or use mushrooms and become cream of mushroom.

Spanish Tomato Basil Soup

Ingredients:

2 cups chicken broth
2 cups of chopped tomato
3 once of tomato paste

4-6 leaves of fresh basil
1-2 cloves of garlic minced
2 tablespoon chopped onion
1/4 tablespoon dried oregano sea salt and pepper

Directions:

Puree all ingredients in a blender. Pour into a saucepan and heat to boil. Simmer for fifteen to twenty minutes. Serve hot, garnish with fresh basil or parsley.

Mexican Corn Chowder

Ingredients: (serves eight)

8 ears of fresh corn kernels or 1 bag of frozen corn
1 yellow onion, chopped
1 medium bell pepper (chopped)
1-2 garlic cloves
1/2 cup cilantro
3/4 cup lemon juice
1 teaspoon cumin
Dash of cayenne pepper salt to taste
Hot water

Directions:

Set aside 1/2 cup corn kernels for garnish. Put all the ingredients in a blender. Blend until smooth, add water if needed. Before serving, blend in very hot water in 1 to 1 ratio of hot water to soup. Garnish with corn kernels and cilantro.

Meat and fish dish — add some steamed or stir fry vegetables and it's a full meal.

Mexican style cilantro chicken

Ingredients:

100gm cubes or sliced chicken
1 chopped tomato
1/2 cup chicken broth

2 tablespoon lemon juice
Fresh chopped cilantro
1 table spoon chopped onion
1/4 tsp. dried oregano
1 clove minced garlic cayenne pepper to taste pinch of salt

Directions:

Lightly brown the chicken with lemon juice and add spices and chicken broth. When the chicken is cooked thoroughly, add fresh tomatoes and cilantro, cook a few minutes then serve.

Oven baked rosemary chicken

Ingredients:

100 gm. chicken breast
1 Melba toast crumbs
1/4 cup chicken broth
3 tablespoon lemon juice
1/2 teaspoon rosemary
1/4 teaspoon onion powder
1/4 teaspoon garlic powder
Pinch of lemon zest Dash of salt and pepper

Directions

Marinate chicken in the lemon juice, salt and rosemary. Mix spices and melba toast crumbles together and coat the chicken with the spice mix. Then add broth. Bake the chicken at 350 for about 15-20 minutes. Sprinkle chicken with lemon juice, salt and pepper to taste.

Fish with Herbs

Ingredients

100gm of white fish
2 tablespoon lemon juice
1 clove crushed garlic
1 tablespoon chopped onion Dill, oregano or thyme pinch of parsley

Directions

Sauté' fish in lemon juice with a little water then add onion, garlic and fresh herbs. Garnish with chopped parsley.

Desert

Tangerine and blood orange pops

1/2 cup fresh lemon juice
1/4 cup lime juice
2.5 cup fresh tangerine juice
3 tangerine, peeled
1 Tablespoon agave or 1/2 tsp. stevia

Honeydew melon pops

4 cups diced ripe honeydew melon
1/3 cup plain soy yogurt juices of 3 limes

1 tablespoon of honey or agave

Combine the ingredient in the blender, fill the ice pop molds with the mixture, insert the sticks, freeze for 6 hours, this will make 8 6oz pops

Nutritional Supplements

Supplements help provide the body with the nutritional elements it needs for maintaining optimal performance. As a basic approach to supplementation, be sure to include high-potency antioxidants and minerals as well as mercury-free fish oils as an abundant source of omega-3 fatty acids.

For more advanced and preventive supplementation, take:

1. Digestive enzymes with each meal to aid digestion and absorption.
2. Probiotics (a source of healthy intestinal bacteria) to improve intestinal protection and function.
3. Fiber with meals to slow down absorption of sugars in food, to feed healthy intestinal bacteria, to prevent constipation and to help the detoxification process.

4. Detoxification supplements such as high dose vitamin C, amino acids, milk thistle, turmeric, broccoli extract, and alpha lipoic acid.

Week 5 — Adding Exercise to Your Daily Routine

Everybody knows it is important to exercise. You may have been too tired or not motivated to exercise in the past. Now that you have more energy with the hormone treatment, it is time to make a commitment to get physically active. It takes an effective approach in order to gain its benefits.

1. Criteria for Effective Exercise:

   a. Duration: at least twenty to thirty minutes, but not longer than an hour.

   b. Frequency: at least three times a week.

   c. Intensity: increase your heart rate to 80 percent of your target heart rate, which is 220 minus your age.

   d. If your exercise pattern does not meet these three criteria, your body will not be able to reap the full benefits of exercise.

2. Types of Exercise

   a. Aerobics: such as brisk walking, jogging, playing tennis, swimming, treadmill, or bicycling. This form of exercise is beneficial for the cardiovascular system because the heart has to pump faster. It also transports more oxygen and nutrients throughout the body, especially the brain, thus preventing age-related memory loss.

   b. Weight training: such as lifting weights. This form of exercise helps to build muscle mass, which helps to burn body fat off, and improves body composition.

   c. Relaxing exercise: such as yoga, tai chi and walking. This form of exercise combines deep breathing and muscle stretching, which helps with relaxation, oxygenation and flexibility.

d.   The best exercise is a combination of all three above. You can start by deep breathing and stretching for ten minutes, followed by jogging or any other form of aerobic exercise for 20 to 30 minutes, then deep breathing and stretching for another ten minutes as a cool down. The warm up and cool down phases are essential to help the muscles prepare for and recover from the exertion of exercising.

3.   The Benefits of Regular Exercise

a.   Improves one's energy production, vitality, and sense of well-being.

b.   Helps the body to lose fat, builds muscle tone, and increases physical strength and endurance.

c.   Reduces cardiovascular diseases and improves blood circulation.

d.   Lowers blood pressure and cholesterol levels.

e.   Improves bone density and helps to prevent osteoporosis.

f.   Improves insulin sensitivity, reduces blood sugar, and helps to prevent diabetes and obesity.

g.   Improves brain function and memory, and helps to prevent senile dementia

h.   Increases the level of endorphins, which helps to maintain positive moods.

i.   Reduce stress and stress-related diseases. Relax the body and mind.

j.   Improve the immune system, thereby reducing the incidence and severity of colds and influenzas.

k.   Reduce insomnia.

l.   Increases the body's natural production of human growth hormone, helping to reverse or slow down the aging process.

4.   The key to making exercise a part of your lifestyle is to motivate yourself by thinking of its benefits and finding a routine that you will do regularly.

5. Exercise daily if possible. Keep a daily log of your exercise. Once it becomes a habit it is very easy to keep. Motivate yourself by finding an exercise partner or rewarding yourself with something you enjoy.

6. This week, we are also going to do another blood test to assess your hormone status, and screen for heavy metals and certain vitamins and minerals.

Week 6 — Toxin Avoidance, Detoxification, and Reevaluation

Helping the body detoxify is an essential part of maintaining our health. An important first step is to avoid toxins in the environment.

Check your kitchen, bathroom, laundry room, medicine cabinet, garage, and storage places. Throw away pesticides, fungicides, harsh environmental unfriendly cleaning solutions and detergents, aluminum containing deodorants and antacids, aluminum foil, aluminum canned-foods and cookware made of aluminum. Do not use plastic food wrap, thin plastic containers or Styrofoam. Check the ingredients in your cosmetics, shampoos, hair dyes and toothpaste; if you see methylparaban, benzene, sodium lauryl sulfate, chlorofluorocarbons, ammonia, or the artificial colors red/yellow/blue, it is time to replace them with products made of natural ingredients. You can usually find them in health food stores.

If you have allergies and your bedroom carpet is old and thick, change it to wood or tile. At least get a HEPA air filter if you cannot replace them right away. If your bathroom and kitchen are damp and dirty, you need to clean them well and improve the ventilation.

If you have not cleaned the air ducts in your house in over seven years, then it is time to get them cleaned.

This week is also the week of re-evaluation. Most of my patients on their return appointment report feeling a lot better already. The common issues I encounter at this stage are insufficient energy, or the inability to lose weight. This may be due to adrenal fatigue, chronic fatigue syndrome, metabolic syndrome, toxin overload, heavy metal toxicity, depression, and leaky gut or food sensitivities.

At this stage, the treatment will depend on each person's unique health issues. The modality we use at this time may include gut healing, detoxification, supplements for adrenal recovery or a weight loss program.

For those improved already, continue your healthy diet, exercise, nutritional supplements, and detoxification so you can reap more benefits.

Week 7 — Unleash Your Subconscious Power

This week, we are going to work on our subconscious mind and our spirituality. We also want to put more joy in our life.

1. Set a time for meditation and creative visualization. The best time is in the morning when you first get up or at night before you go to bed. Create a place you can go without being interrupted. For details about how to do meditation and creative visualization, please see pages 209-213.

2. Set a time to read spiritual books or pray. In the morning or at night are both good times. For Christians, reading the Bible should be a daily routine. For others I suggest the book *50 Spiritual Classics* which will give you a good selection of spiritual titles to browse.

3. Create a place you can go to relax or meditate, at work and at home.

4. Find enjoyable things (people or movie, etc.) that make you laugh.

5. Write down five enjoyable activities and do them regularly. For example, nice soothing massage, relaxing music, a beach walk, a warm bath, etc.

My thirteen year old son and I have a nightly routine. He loves to get a massage at night to put him to sleep. What I usually do is to give him a massage around his neck, back and shoulder and using the technique of progressive relaxation, by saying things like this: "take a deep breath, inhale through your nose and exhale through your mouth. Squeeze your neck then relax, now take another deep breath, squeeze your arms then relax, now take another deep breath and squeeze your shoulders then relax and take another deep breath, squeeze your legs then relax. Now your body is totally relaxed."

After this, I will put my hand on his lower abdomen, where the first and second chakras are, massage in a circular motion, and say: "You are loved by your family and friends, you are safe and secure. You are a good student and in the future, you will have a successful career and a happy family." Then I move to the third chakra, "You know you are smart and good looking. You take good care of yourself by eating more fruits and vegetables. You also know your responsibilities and can perform them well." then I move my hands to his heart chakra and say, "You feel your emotions, if there is anger, frustration, fear or sadness, let it pass through you. Focus on solution of the problem. There is no need for anxiety or fear, and you can feel the happiness and joy. You can also sense other people's feelings." The next one is the throat chakra, and I will put my hand there and say "You know how to express your feelings and communicate well. You can stand up for yourself." Then I put my hand on top of his head, again massaging his scalp in a circular motion, and say, "You are a precious and holy child of God. God loves you and gives you so many talents. You will use those talents well and always know how to connect to God by using your intuition." The whole process only takes less than ten minutes and he usually is fast sleep. I am hoping all my suggestions go to his subconscious mind and improve his subtle energy and spirit.

Daily Planning

Week 8 — Putting It All Together

An ancient Chinese proverb says: "We are born similar, but different habits set us apart." It is true that different habits make us different people. That is why we need good habits. Once an activity becomes a habit, it is easier to follow through on it more consistently.

The famous Chinese scholar, Master Zhang, said: "I review my behavior three times a day." Routinely evaluating our own behavior gives us more insight into who we are and what we are setting as our priorities. An honest evaluation will help us become better people and work more effectively.

It is a good habit to plan our daily lives and evaluate our behavior daily. Here is an example of daily planning:

List and Prioritize Daily Tasks:

1.
2.
3.
4.
5.
6.
7.
8.
9.
10.

Daily review: You can develop questions to ask yourself on a daily basis.

What did I do today for my body?

- Did I eat healthy meals?
- Did I take my supplements?
- Did I drink eight glasses of water?
- Did I exercise sufficiently?

What did I do today for my mind and spirit?

- Did I read the Bible or other spiritual books?
- Did I meditate or pray?
- Did I do something to help another person(s)?
- Did I do something to make myself and other people laugh?
- Did I find three things for which to be grateful?

Based on this kind of daily planning, we can also develop weekly, monthly, and yearly planning. It is a bit like planning for a trip. The more details you plan in advance, the more quickly you will arrive at your destination and the more you will enjoy your trip.

Summary

Emotional and spiritual health provides the foundation for healthy aging. This is not easy to achieve if you are suffering emotionally, or are not in touch with a purpose for your life. Healthy aging takes discipline, determination, and effort. Healthy aging is a choice and only you can decide to engage in what it takes to achieve this desirable condition. Is it worth it? Oh, yes. It's you and your entire being — your vitality!

Recommended Reading

Amen, Daniel, M.D. Change Your Brain, Change Your Life. Three River Press,

Arpaia, Joseph, M.D. Tibetan Wisdom for Western Life. Beyond Words Publishing, 1999.

Bruce H Lipton, Ph.D. The biology of Belief. Hay House,2005

Butler-Bowdon, Tom. 50 Spiritual Classics: Timeless Wisdom from 50 Great Books on Inner Discovery, Enlightenment and Purpose. Nicholas Brealey Publishing, 2005.

Caddy, Eileen. God Spoke to Me. Findhorn Press, 1971. Candace Pert, Molecules of Emotion, Touch stone, 1999

Colborn Theo, Dianne Dumanoski, and John Peterson Myers. Our Stolen Future: Are We Threatening Our Fertility, Intelligence, and Survival? — A Scientific Detective Story. Plume, 1997.

Cornbleet, Jennifer. Raw Food Made Easy for 1 or 2 People. Book Publishing Company, 2005.

Dyer, Wayne, Ph.D. 10 Secrets for Success and Inner Peace. Hay House, Inc., 2002. Gawain, Shakti. Creative Visualization Meditations. New World Library, 2002. Gittleman, Ann Louise and Sears, Barry, Ph.D. The Fat Flush Plan. McGraw-Hill, 2002.

Hay, Louise. You Can Heal Your Life Affirmation Kit. 2005. Hunt, Valerie. Infinite Mind. Malibu Publishing Company, 1997.

Hyman, Mark, M.D. The UltraMind Solution: Fix Your Broken Brain By Healing Your Body First. Scribner, 2008.

Jack Kornfield The Wise Heart. Bantam Books, 2009

MacDonald Baker, Sidney, M.D. Detoxification and Healing: The Key to Optimal Health. McGraw-Hill, 2003

Mona Lisa Schulz M.D. Ph.D. The Intuitive Advisor, Hay House, 2009

Northrup, Christiane, M.D. The Wisdom of Menopause: Creating Physical and Emotional Health and Healing During the Change, 2nd ed. Bantam, 2006.

Null, Gary, Ph.D. Gary Null's Power Aging. New American Library Trade, 2004.

Prager, Dennis. Happiness Is a Serious Problem: A Human Nature Repair Manual. Harper Collins, 1998.

Rogers, Sherry, M.D. Wellness Against All Odds. Prestige Publications, 1994.

Sears, Barry, Ph.D. The Age-Free Zone. Collins Living, 2000.

Shames, Richard, M.D., and Karilee Shames. Thyroid Power: Ten Steps to Total Health. Collins Living, 2002.

Roizen, Michael, M.D., Oz, Mehmet, M.D. You: Staying Young: The Owner's Manual for Extending Your Warranty. Free Press, 2007.

Somers, Suzanne. Breakthrough: Eight Steps to Wellness. Crown, 2008.

Sinatra, Steven, M.D. Lower Your Blood Pressure in Eight Weeks: A Revolutionary Program for a Longer, Healthier Life. Ballantine Books, 2003.

Sinatra, Steven, M.D., James Roberts, and Zucker, Martin. Reverse Heart Disease Now: Stop Deadly Cardiovascular Plaque Before It's Too Late. Wiley, 2008.

Tolle, Eckhart. The Power of Now: A Guide To Spiritual Enlightenment. Namaste Publishing, 1990.

Warren, Rick. The Purpose Driven Life. Zondervan, 2002.

Weil, Andrew, M.D. Healthy Aging: A Lifelong Guide to Your Well-being. Anchor, 2007.

Wilson, James, N.D. Adrenal Fatigue: The 21st Century Stress Syndrome. Smart Publications, 2002.

References

1. Ferrara A, Karter AJ, Ackerson LM, et al. Hormone replacement therapy is associated with better glycemic control in women with type 2 diabetes: The Northern California Kaiser Permanente Diabetes Registry. Diabetes Care. 2001;24(7):1144-1150.

2. Seely EW, Walsh BW, Gerhard MD, Williams GH. Estradiol with or without progesterone and ambulatory blood pressure in postmenopausal women. Hypertension. 1999;33(5):1190-1194.

3. Wagner JD. Rationale for hormone replacement in atherosclerosis prevention. J Reprod Med. 2000;45(3 suppl):245-258.

4. Tang MX, Jacobs D, Stern Y, et al. Effect of oestrogen during menopause on risk and age onset of Alzheimer's disease. Lancet. 1996;348(9025):429-432.

5. Wise PM, Dubal DB, Wilson ME, Rau SW, Bottner M. Minireview: neuroprotective effects of estrogen-new insight into mechanism of action. Endocrinology. 2001;142(3):969-973.

6. Snow KK, Seddon JM. Age related eye diseases: impact of hormone replacement therapy, and reproductive and other risk factors. Int J Fertil Womens Med. 2000;45(5): 301-313.

7. Writing Group for the Women's Health Initiative Investigators. Risks and benefits of estrogen plus progestin in healthy postmenopausal women: Principal results from the Women's Health Initiative randomized controlled trial. JAMA. 2002;288(3):321-333.

8. Yates J, Barrett-Connor E, Barlas S, Chen YT, Miller PD, Siris ES. Rapid loss of hip fracture protection after estrogen cessation: evidence from the National Osteoporosis Risk Assessment. Obstet Gynecol. 2004;103(3):440-446.

9. Chlebowski RT, Hendrix SL, Langer RD, et al. Influence of estrogen plus progestin on breast cancer and mammography in healthy postmenopausal women: the Women's Health Initiative randomized trial. JAMA. 2003;289(24):3243-3253.

10. Schairer C, Adami HO, Hoover R, Persson I. Cause specific mortality in women receiving hormone replacement therapy. Epidemiology. 1997;8(1):59-65.

11. Vassilopoulou — Sellin R, Asmar L, Hortobagyi GN, et al. Estrogen replacement therapy after localized breast cancer: Clinical outcome of 319 women followed prospectively. J Clin Oncol. 1999;17(5): 1482-1487.

12. Vassilopoulou-Sellin R, Cohen DS, Hortobagyi GN, et al. Estrogen replacement therapy for menopausal women with a history of breast carcinoma: Results of a 5 year, prospective study. Cancer. 2002;95(9):1817-1826.

13. Meurer LN, Lena S. Cancer recurrence and mortality in women using hormone replacement therapy after breast cancer: Meta-analysis. J Fam Pract. 2002;51(12): 1056-1062.

14. Pasqualini JR, Gelly C, Nguyen BL, Vella C. Importance of estrogen sulfates in breast cancer. J Steroid Biochem. 1989;34(1-6):155-163.

15. Jefcoate CR, Liehr JC, Santen RJ, et al. Tissue-specific synthesis and oxidative metabolism of estrogens. J Natl Cancer Inst Monogr. 2000;27:95-112.

16. Chang M, Zhang F, Shen L, et al. Inhibition of glutathione S-transferase activity by the quinoid metabolites of equine estrogens. Chem Res Toxicol. 1998;11(7):758-765.

17. Chen Y, Shen L, Zhang F, et al. The equine estrogen metabolite 4- hydroxye- quilenin cause DNA single-strand breaks and oxidation of DNA bases in vitro. Chem Res Toxicol. 1998;(11):1105-1111.

18. Cowan LD, Gordis L, Tonascia JA, Jones GS. Breast cancer incidence in women with a history of progesterone deficiency. Am J Epidemiol. 1981;114(2):209-217.

19. Barrat J, de Lignieres B, Marpeau L, et al. The in vivo effect of the local administration of progesterone on the mitotic activity of human ductal breast tissue. Results of a pilot study. J Gynecol Obstet Biol Reprod. 1990;19(3):269-274.

20. Formby B, Wiley TS. Progesterone inhibits growth and induces apoptosis in breast cancer cells: Inverse effects on Bcl-2 and p53. Ann Clin Lab Sci. 1998;28(6): 360-369.

21. Formby B, Wiley TS. Bcl-2, survivin and variant CD44 v7-v10 are downregualted and p53 is upregulated in breast cancer cells by progesterone: Inhibition of cell growth and induction of apoptosis. Mol Cell Biochem. 1999;202(1-2):53-61.

22. Leo JC, Wang SM, Guo CH, et al. Gene regulation profile reveals consistent anticancer properties of progesterone in hormone-independent breast cancer cells transfected with progesterone receptor. Int J Cancer. 2005;117(4):561-568.

23. Clarkson TB. Progesterone and cardiovascular disease. A critical review. J Reprod Med. 1999;44(2 suppl):180-184.

24. The writing group for the PEPI trial. Effects of estrogen or estrogen/progestin regimen on heart disease risk factors in postmenopausal women. The PEPI trial. JAMA. 1995;273(3):199-208.

25. Rosano GM; Webb CM, Chierchia S, et al. Natural progesterone, but not medroxyprogesterone acetate, enhances the beneficial effect of estrogen on exercise induced

myocardial ischemia in postmenopausal women. J Am Coll Cardiol. 2000;36(7):2154-2159.

26. Dimitrakakis C, Zhou J, Wang J, et al. A physiological role for testosterone in limiting estrogenic stimulation of the breast. Menopause. 2003;10(4):274-276.

27. Ando S, De Amicis F, Rago V, et al. Breast cancer: From estrogen to androgen receptor. Mol Cell Endocrinol. 2002;193(1-2):121-128.

28. Sanchez-Barcelo EJ, Cos S, Fernandz R, Mediavilla MD. Melatonin and mammary cancer: A short review. Endocr Relat Cancer. 2003;10(2):153-159.

29. Anisimov VN. The light-dark regimen and cancer development. Neuro Endocrinol Lett. 2002;Jul;23(suppl 2): 28-36.

30. Chen FP, Lee N, Soong YK, Huang KE. Comparison of transdermal and oral estrogen-replacement therapy: Effects on cardiovascular risk factors. Menopause. 2001;8 (5):347-352.

31. Scarabin PY, Alhenc-Gelas M, Plu-Bureau G, Taisne P, Agher R, Aiach M. Effects of oral and transdermal estrogen/progesterone regimens on blood coagulation and fibrinolysis in postmenopausal women. A randomized control trial. Artherioscler Thromb Vasc Biol. 1997;17(11): 3071-3078.

32. Studd JW, Smith RN. Oestradiol and testosterone implants. Baillieres Clin Endocrinol Metab. 1993;7(1):203-223.

33. Greenblatt RB, Studd JW (eds). Oestrogen therapy and the menopausal syndrome. The Menopause. Clin Obstet Gynecol. 1977;4(1):31-48.

34. Davelaar EM, Gerretsen G, Relyveld J. No increase in the incidence of breast carcinoma with subcutaneous administration of estradiol. Ned Tijdschr Geneeskd. 1991;135(14):613-615.

35. Notelovitz M, Johnston M, Smith S, Kitchens C. Metabolic and hormonal effects of 25mg and 50mg 17 beta-estradiol implants in surgically menopausal women. Obstet Gynecol. 1987;70(5):749-754.

36. Farrish E, Fletcher CD, Hart DM, Azzawi FA, Abdalla HI, Gray CE. The effects of hormone implants on serum lipoprotein and steroid hormones bilaterally oophorectomised women. Acta Endocrinol (Copenh). 1984;106(1):116-20.

37. Burger HG, Hailes J, Menelaus M, Nelson J, Hudson B, Balazs N. The management of persistent menopausal symptoms with oestradiol-testosterone implants: clinical, lipid and hormone result. Maturitas. 1982;6(4):351-358.

38. Studd J, Savvas M, Waston N, Garnett T, Fogelman I, Cooper D. The relationship between plasma estradiol and the increase in bone density in postmenopausal women after treatment with subcutaneous hormone implants. Am J Obstet Gynecol. 1990;163(5 part 1): 1474-1479.

39. Montgomery JC, Appleby L, Brincat M, et al. Effect of oestrogen and testosterone implants on psychological disorders in the climacteric. Lancet. 1987;1 (8628):297-299.

40. Bachmann G, Bancroft J, Braunstein G, et al. Female androgen insufficiency: The Princeton consensus statement on definition, classification, and assessment. Fertil Steril. 2002;77(4):660-665.

41. Tutera G. You Don't have to Live with It! Scottsdale, AZ: SottoPelle; 2003:72.

42. Statin P, Lumme S, Tenkanen L, et al, High levels of circulating testosterone are not associated with increased prostate cancer risk: A pooled prospective study. Int J Cancer. 2004;108(3):418-424.

43. Rhoden EL, Morgentaler A. Testosterone replacement therapy in hypogonadal men at high risk for prostate cancer:

Results of 1 year of treatment in men with prostatic intraepithelial neoplasia. J Urol. 2004;170(6 Pt 1);2348-2351.

44. Snyder PJ, Peachey H, Berlin JA, et al. Effects of testosterone replacement in hypogonadal men. J Clin Endocrinol Metab. 2000;85(8):2670-2677.

45. Cohen PG. The hypogonadal-obesity cycle: role of aromatase in modulating the testosterone-estradiol shunt — a major factor in the genesis of morbid obesity. Med Hypotheses. 1999;52(1):49-51.

46. Cooper MA, Ritchie EC. Testosterone replacement therapy for anxiety. Am J Psychiatry. 2000;157(11):1884.

47. Makinen J, Jarvisalo MJ, Pollanen P, et al. Increased carotid atherosclerosis in andropausal middle-aged men. J Am Coll Cardiol. 2005;45(10):1603-1608.

48. Margolese HC. The male menopause and mood: Testosterone decline and depression in the aging male — Is there a link? J Geriatr Psychiatry Neurol. 2000;13(2):93-101.

49. Hak AE, Witteman JC, de Jong FH, Geerlings MI, Hofman A, Pols HA. Low levels of endogenous androgens increase the risk of atherosclerosis in elderly men: The Rotterdam Study. J Clin Endocrinol Metab. 2002;87(8):3632-3639.

50. Wang C, Swerdloff RS, Iranmanesh A, et al. Testosterone improves sexual function, mood, and muscle strength and body composition parameters in hypogonadal men. J Clin Endocrinol Metab. 2000;85(8):2839-2853.

51. Rosano G, Leonardo F, Pagnotta P, et al. Acute anti-ischemic effect of testosterone in men with coronary artery disease. Circulation. 1999;99(13):1666-1670.

52. Stellato RK, Feldman HA, Hamdy O, Horton ES, McKinlay JB. Testosterone, sex hormone-binding globulin, and the development of type 2 diabetes in middle-aged men:

prospective results from the Massachusetts male aging study. Diabetes Care. 2000;23(4):490-494.

53. Dhindsa S, Prabhakar S, Sethi M, Bandyopadhyay A, Chaudhuri A, Dandona P. Frequent occurrence of hypogonadotropic hypogonadism in type II diabetes. J Clin Endocrinol Metab. 2004;89:5462-5468.

54. Moffat SD, Zonderman AB, Metter EJ, Blackman MR, Harman SM, Resnick SM. Longitudinal assessment of serum free testosterone concentration predicts memory performance and cognitive status in elderly men. J Clin Endocrinol Metab. 2002;87(11):5001-5007.

55. Gouras GK, Xu H, Gross RS, et al. Testosterone reduces neuronal secretion of Alzheimer's beta amyloid peptides. Proc Natl Acad Sci USA. 2000;97(3):1202-1205.

56. Eastell R, Boyle IT, Compston J, et al. Management of male osteoporosis: report of the UK Consensus group. QJM. 1998;91(2):71-92.

57. AACE Thyroid Task Force. American Association of Clinical Endocrinologists medical guidelines for clinical practice for the evaluation and treatment of hyperthyroidism and hypothyroidism. Endocr Pract. 2002;8(6):457-469.

58. Brucker DF. Effects of environmental synthetic chemicals on the thyroid function. Thyroid. 1998;8(9):827-856.

59. Colquhoun J. Why I changed my mind about water fluoridation. Perspect Biol Med. 1997;41(1):29-44.

60. Baisier WV, Hertoghe J, W. Eeckhaut W. Thyroid insufficiency. Is thyroxine the only valuable drug? J Nutr Environ Med. 2001;11(3):159-166.

61. Levin HS, Rodnitzky RL. Behavioral effects of organophosphate pesticides in man. Clin Tox. 1976;9(3):391-405.

62. Feldman RG, Ricks NL, Baker EL, Neuropsychological effects of industrial toxins: A review. Am J Ind Med. 1980;1(2):211-227.

63. White R, Jobling S, Hoare SA, Sumpter JP, Parker MG, et al. Environmentally persistent alkylphenolic compounds are estrogenic. Endocrinology. 1994;135(1):175-182.

64. Shenker BJ, TL Guo TL, Shapiro IM. Low level methylmercury exposure causes human T cells to undergo apoptosis: evidence of mitochondrial dysfunction. Environ Res. 1998;77:149-59.

65. DeSouza Queiroz ML, Pena SC, Salles TSI, de Capitani EM, Olalla Saad ST. Abnormal antioxidant system in erythrocytes of mercury exposed workers. Human & Exp Toxicol. 1998;17:225-230.

66. Ngim CH, Foo SC, Boey KW, JeyaratnamJ. Chronic neurobehavioral effects of elemental mercury in dentists. Brit J Indust Med. 1992;49:782-790.

67. Solonen JT, Seppanen K, Nyyssonen K, et al. Intake of mercury from fish, lipid peroxidation, and the risk of myocardial infarction and coronary, cardiovascular, and early death in eastern Finnish men. Circulation. 1995;91(3):645-655.

68. Perl DP, Brody AR. Alzheimer's disease: X-ray spectrometric evidence of aluminum accumulation in neurofibrillary tangle-bearing neurons. Sci. 1980;208(4441):297-299.

69. Folsom AR, Aleksic N, Catellier D, et al. C-reactive protein and incident coronary heart disease in the atherosclerosis risk in communities (ARIC) study. Am Heart J. 2002;144(2):233-238.

70. Futterman LG, Lemberg L. High-sensitive C-reactive protein is the most effective prognostic measurement of acute coronary events. Am J Crit Care. 2002;11(5): 482-486.

71. Clarke, R, Daly L, Robinson K, et al. Hyperhomocysteine: An independent factor for vascular disease. N Eng J Med, 1991;324:1149-1155.

72. Motoyama T, Sano H, Fukuzaki H. Oral magnesium supplementation in patients with essential hypertension. Hypertension. 1989;13:227-232.

73. Cantor KP, Lynch CF, Hildesheim ME, et al. Drinking water source and chlorination by-products. I. Risk of bladder cancer. Epidemiology. 1998;9:21-28.

74. Porta M, Malats N, Jariod M, et al. Serum concentration of organochlorine compounds and K-ras mutations in exocrine pancreatic cancer. PANKRAS II Study Group. Lancet. 1999;354(9196):2125-2130.

75. DeFronzo RA, Ferranni E. Insulin resistance: A multifaceted syndrome responsible for NIDDM, obesity, hypertension, dyslipidemia, and atherosclerotic cardiovascular disease. Diabetes Care. 1991:14(3):173-194.

Index

Acetylcholine, 18, 190, 192, 193, 229
ACTH, adrenocorticotropic hormone, 8
Acupuncture, 150
Adrenal fatigue, xi, xx, xxi, xxii, 46, 47, 49, 53, 60, 64, 79, 80, 82, 83, 84, 88, 89, 90, 91, 92, 100, 101, 104, 252, 259
Adrenal gland/hormones, xxi, xxii, 9, 17, 46, 47, 60, 79, 80, 81, 82, 84, 85, 88, 89, 90, 91, 94, 103, 189, 192
Aerobic exercise, 107, 172, 194, 228, 237, 251
Aging, i, iii, v, ix, xi, xii, xiv, xvii, xx, xxiii, 1, 5, 6, 7, 8, 9, 10, 11, 12, 22, 23, 54, 59, 64, 65, 68, 70, 74, 90, 94, 105, 106, 116, 118, 120, 129, 136, 138, 180, 181, 182, 183, 184, 186, 193, 195, 209, 213, 226, 227, 228, 229, 231, 242, 251, 256, 258, 259, 266, 267
Aldosterone, 80, 81, 82
Alpha lipoic acid, 10, 225, 229, 250

Aluminum, 162, 163, 165, 221, 252, 268
Alzheimer's disease, xi, xvii, 5, 11, 22, 59, 73, 189, 213, 261, 268
Amino acids, 105, 106, 107, 113, 118, 129, 134, 137, 138, 148, 161, 166, 167, 168, 174, 190, 191, 195, 227, 239, 250
Androgen, 45, 264, 265
Andropause/andropausal, x, 67
  testosterone deficiency, x, 44, 63, 65, 67
Antibiotics, 3, 136, 138, 139, 145, 147
Antidepressants, xviii, 15, 41, 42, 44, 49, 53, 70, 191, 193, 194, 228
Armour thyroid, 94, 101
Aromatase enzyme, 26
Aromatase inhibitor, 68, 69, 78
Arthritis, 3, 5, 8, 11, 19, 59, 99, 109, 138, 213
Atherosclerosis, 5, 11, 59, 70, 96, 118, 120, 159, 212, 213, 215, 224, 227, 261, 266, 268
Atrophy, 55, 77

Brain, 192
  testicular, 77
Autoimmune disease, 99,
  159, 235
Beauty, xiii, 179, 186
  self-esteem, xiii, 198, 202
Benign prostate
  hypertrophy, 77
Beta carotene, 216, 222
Bio-identical hormone
  replacement therapy, 44,
  59, 64, 66
Bleeding, 35, 41, 49, 61, 62,
  120, 140
  fibroids, 62
  heavy, xviii, 59, 62
  pellet implants, x, 29, 33,
  41, 44, 52, 76, 78, 194
Blood pressure, 18, 22, 25,
  34, 50, 73, 80, 81, 82, 121,
  122, 213, 215, 216, 226,
  251, 258, 261
Blood sugar (glucose), 22,
  80, 81, 86, 91, 100, 114,
  124, 126, 214, 224, 226,
  251
Bone mineral density
  (BMD), 229
Bowel, 169, 171, 173, 219
  irritable, 159
Brain, xiii, xiv, xxiii, 8, 9, 12,
  18, 19, 70, 80, 81, 82, 83,
  85, 87, 96, 98, 105, 107,
  120, 155, 175, 176, 187,
  188, 189, 190, 192, 193,
  194, 195, 198, 201, 203,
  212, 226, 227, 228, 229,
  235, 239, 250, 251, 257

Breast cancer, ix, x, xxiii, 15,
  16, 19, 23, 24, 25, 26, 34,
  55, 56, 57, 58, 62, 64, 77,
  151, 168, 202, 218, 219,
  262, 263, 264
  bio-identical pellet
  therapy, 44, 59, 64, 66
  prevention, x, 57
  progesterone, 16, 60, 194
C0-Q10, 167, 216, 229
Coronary artery disease
  see
  cardiovascular/corona
  ry artery/heart
  disease, 266
Cabbage, 58, 115, 120, 128,
  168, 172, 174, 221, 245
Calcium, 102, 121, 122, 144,
  162, 212, 230, 231
Cancer, xiv, xvii, xxiii, 3, 5,
  19, 22, 23, 24, 25, 26, 27,
  50, 55, 56, 57, 58, 61, 62,
  69, 82, 121, 123, 141, 155,
  156, 157, 159, 168, 180,
  211, 213, 217, 218, 219,
  220, 221, 222, 262, 263,
  264, 265, 269
Candida, xii, xx, 139, 142,
  144, 145, 177, 236
Carbohydrates, 86, 113, 114,
  115, 124, 126, 127, 128,
  131, 134, 135, 145, 221,
  223, 243
Cardiovascular/coronary
  artery heart disease, xiv,
  211, 213, 215
Chelation therapy, 161
  DMPS, 160, 161, 162, 177
  DMSA, 160, 162

Chemical sensitivity, 176
Chinese, 150, 175, 201, 254
  herbs, 47, 78, 85, 89, 91,
  102, 127, 131, 137, 143,
  148, 161, 174, 183, 225,
  229, 239, 248, 249
Chlorides, 138, 163
Chlorine, 97, 98, 102, 126,
  154
Cholesterol, 70, 75, 96, 98,
  99, 118, 125, 131, 212,
  213, 215, 217, 223, 224,
  225, 226, 251
Chromium, 122, 225
Chronic fatigue syndrome,
  99, 159
Coenzyme Q10, 167, 225
Colon, 121, 135, 165, 171,
  172, 217, 218, 219, 220
Compounding pharmacies,
  38
Constipation, 80, 96, 98, 101,
  102, 103, 122, 125, 140,
  145, 146, 147, 171, 172,
  219, 225, 234, 249
Cortisol, 17, 58, 60, 80, 81,
  82, 84, 90, 91, 92, 103,
  192, 193, 194, 216, 226
Cortisone, 80, 141, 193
Creams (hormones), xix, 15,
  28, 48
CRP (C-reactive protein),
  213, 268
Cruciferous vegetables, 58,
  128, 167, 168, 174
Dementia, xiv, 22, 25, 31, 54,
  59, 73, 158, 226, 227, 251
Depression, 5, 18, 34, 39, 43,
  44, 49, 50, 53, 57, 63, 66,

70, 73, 77, 82, 83, 91, 96,
98, 99, 101, 103, 121, 150,
158, 190, 191, 192, 193,
198, 199, 235, 253, 266
Detoxification, xiv, xxii,
  xxiii, 5, 10, 24, 57, 58, 68,
  102, 113, 120, 122, 125,
  127, 135, 140, 150, 158,
  160, 162, 165, 166, 167,
  168, 169, 173, 174, 177,
  214, 216, 217, 221, 222,
  225, 226, 249, 250, 252,
  253, 258
DHEA, 17, 23, 26, 46, 47,
  58, 60, 80, 82, 84, 90, 91,
  228
Diabetes, xiv, 3, 4, 11, 12,
  22, 25, 59, 73, 77, 78, 81,
  82, 83, 91, 96, 99, 106,
  107, 109, 122, 123, 124,
  213, 215, 223, 224, 228,
  236, 251, 261, 266, 267,
  269
  insulin resistance, xiv, 25,
    46, 73, 99, 115, 124, 223
  laboratory testing, 60
  testosterone and insulin,
    x, 71
Diet, xi, xii, xiv, 4, 5, 21, 58,
  86, 91, 93, 102, 107, 113,
  116, 118, 126, 127, 128,
  129, 130, 131, 137, 140,
  143, 145, 147, 148, 164,
  168, 176, 183, 185, 195,
  215, 221, 225, 227, 230,
  242, 243, 253
  anti-inflammation diet,
    215
  healthy aging diet, 227

weight loss diet, xii, 127
Digestive, 11, 142, 234, 249
   Enzyme, 11, 96, 114, 134,
      136, 142, 147, 148
   tract/system, 106, 114, 202
Dizziness/dizzy, 83, 167,
   176
DMPS chelation, 177
DMSA chelation, 161
Duodenum, 134, 135
EDTA chelation, 162
Electromagnetic fields, 174
Emotion, 192, 203, 257
Endorphins (beta), 215, 228,
   251
Environmental toxins, 10,
   57, 94, 97, 101, 102, 104,
   140, 165, 178, 213, 217,
   225, 226
Enzymes, 11, 21, 113, 114,
   119, 121, 125, 128, 129,
   131, 133, 134, 136, 142,
   162, 166, 167, 168, 217,
   249
Essential amino acids, 118
Essential fatty acids, 86, 116,
   126
Estradiol, xviii, 17, 18, 19,
   21, 23, 24, 25, 34, 36, 38,
   42, 48, 50, 52, 57, 60, 61,
   62, 68, 69, 78, 106, 193,
   261, 264, 265, 266
Estriol, 17
Estrogen dominance, x, 19,
   57, 58, 62, 63
Estrogen-plus-progestin,
   261, 262
   breast cancer, xxiii, 15, 16,
      19, 23, 24, 25, 26, 34,

55, 56, 57, 58, 62, 64,
   77, 151, 168, 202, 218,
   219, 262, 263
   coronary heart disease, 25,
      268
   strokes, 12, 31, 214, 215,
      224
Estrogens, 16, 21, 23, 24, 68,
   262
   estradiol, 16, 18, 19
   estriol, 16
   estrone, 17, 18
Estrone, 17, 21
Exercise, xiv, xx, xxiii, 3, 4,
   6, 12, 15, 25, 37, 58, 63,
   65, 66, 67, 87, 93, 103,
   106, 107, 109, 129, 170,
   172, 173, 176, 186, 194,
   213, 215, 222, 226, 227,
   228, 231, 237, 239, 242,
   250, 251, 252, 253, 255,
   263
   health benefits, 172, 222
FAIS, 45, 46
Fasting insulin values, 224,
   236
Fat, 15, 17, 19, 35, 45, 61,
   63, 68, 73, 77, 78, 81, 89,
   96, 108, 109, 113, 114,
   115, 116, 117, 118, 119,
   127, 128, 129, 134, 135,
   136, 137, 168, 181, 183,
   195, 197, 217, 223, 226,
   244, 250, 251, 257
Fatigue, xxi, xxiii, 15, 22, 39,
   45, 46, 47, 54, 57, 59, 64,
   66, 67, 77, 81, 82, 83, 84,
   86, 88, 90, 91, 95, 101,

103, 119, 126, 139, 145,
150, 158, 176
adrenal, xi, xx, xxi, xxii,
46, 47, 49, 53, 60, 64,
79, 80, 82, 83, 84, 88,
89, 90, 91, 92, 100, 101,
104, 252, 259
chronic, xxiii, 83, 91, 147,
151, 202, 252
Fiber, 58, 86, 89, 102, 114,
115, 124, 125, 127, 128,
131, 136, 140, 147, 171,
172, 173, 174, 217, 221,
222, 225, 249
Fibrinogen, 214, 236
Fibroid tumors, 19, 59, 61,
62
Fibromyalgia syndrome, 177
First-pass liver metabolism
(see liver), 27
Fish oil, 116, 129, 225, 228,
249
Flaxseed oil/fiber/meal, 116,
117, 129
Fluoride, 97, 102, 126, 163
Folate, 58, 168, 216
Folic acid, 119, 144, 166,
214, 216
Food allergies, xx, 97, 100,
128, 133, 136, 142, 143,
145, 147
tests, 97
Free radicals, ix, 5, 9, 10, 88,
120, 127, 157, 166, 167,
181, 182, 212, 217, 221,
222, 225, 226, 227, 229,
231
Oxidative Stress Theory,
ix, 9

Free testosterone, 46, 66, 67,
68, 70, 73, 267
FSH (follicle stimulating
hormone), 9, 36, 46, 59, 60
GABA, 19, 190, 191, 193,
239
Gallbladder, 135
Gamma-linolenic acid
(GLA), 116
Genes, 4, 8, 168
Gene control, ix, 7
Telomeres, ix, 7
GERD, xii, 136, 137
GI Tract, xii, 133, 136, 141,
145, 147, 148, 177
Glucose (see blood sugar),
34, 81, 89, 96, 113, 122,
138, 225
Glutamate, 190, 191
Glycemic index, 115, 126,
127, 131, 223
Glycogen, 135
Goiter, 97, 100, 123
Green tea, 214
Growth hormone, 8, 18, 23,
58, 105, 106, 107, 129,
189, 191, 216, 228, 251
Hair, 7, 19, 39, 48, 61, 67,
93, 94, 99, 103, 123, 159,
162, 164, 165, 175, 181,
184, 221, 234, 252
Hair analysis, 159, 162
Hashimoto's thyroiditis, 97
Headaches, 3, 4, 39, 41, 42,
82, 138, 176
Heart disease, xvii, 3, 11, 12,
31, 73, 99, 123, 212, 220,
223, 258, 263

Heavy metals, xxii, 102, 123, 125, 141, 153, 157, 158, 159, 160, 161, 162, 165, 166, 213, 225, 236, 252

Herbs, 47, 78, 85, 89, 91, 102, 127, 131, 137, 143, 148, 161, 174, 183, 225, 229, 239, 248, 249

HGH (see human growth hormone), 8, 23, 58, 105, 106, 107

High blood pressure (see blood pressure), 70, 122, 216, 226

Homocysteine, 213, 214, 215, 216, 236

Hormone(s), v, ix, x, xi, xiii, xiv, xvii, xviii, xix, xxi, xxii, xxiii, 5, 9, 10, 13, 15, 16, 17, 18, 20, 21, 22, 23, 24, 25, 26, 27, 28, 29, 30, 31, 33, 34, 36, 37, 38, 39, 40, 41, 42, 43, 45, 46, 48, 51, 53, 54, 55, 56, 57, 58, 59, 60, 61, 64, 65, 66, 68, 69, 72, 74, 75, 76, 78, 80, 82, 84, 87, 89, 90, 92, 93, 94, 95, 98, 99, 100, 102, 103, 105, 106, 108, 109, 116, 118, 129, 149, 153, 156, 163, 178, 181, 191, 192, 193, 194, 216, 217, 220, 222, 223, 227, 228, 230, 236, 237, 250, 252, 261, 262, 263, 265, 266

Bio-identical, ix, x, xviii, xix, xx, 15, 16, 20, 21, 24, 25, 27, 29, 30, 33, 38, 42, 43, 44, 48, 53, 54, 56, 59, 64, 65, 66, 72, 74, 75, 76, 78, 90, 92, 94, 102, 106, 149, 178, 194, 230, 237

blood pressure, 18, 22, 25, 34, 50, 73, 80, 81, 121, 122, 213, 215, 216, 226, 251, 261

bones, 18, 42, 54, 74, 105, 106, 118, 121, 122, 130, 157, 162, 215, 230, 231

creams, xix, 15, 21, 28, 48

fibroids, 62

ovary/ovaries, 27

pellet implants, 51

pituitary gland, 36

PMS (premenstrual syndrome), x, 19, 62, 119, 191, 194, 202

Synthetic, ix, 20, 21, 33, 37

Hot flushes/hot flashes, xvii, xviii, 15, 16, 22, 31, 39, 40, 41, 51, 52, 53, 54, 59, 60, 93, 234

HRT (hormone replacement therapy), ix, x, 19, 22, 23, 24, 26, 31, 34, 59, 70, 74, 77

Alzheimer's disease, 59

beneficial/protection, ix, x, 15, 22, 23, 27, 33

blood pressure, 22

bones/osteoporosis/bones, 22

brain, 60

breast cancer risk, 23, 26

cardiovascular/coronary, 268

creams (hormone), xix,
  15, 28, 48
depression, 22
estradiol, 18, 19
estriol, 17
estrogen, 23, 24
estrone, 17, 18
heart disease, 25, 31
interstitial cystitis, 47, 49
menopause/postmenopaus
  e, ix, xviii, xix, xxi, xxii,
  15, 16, 17, 18, 20, 22,
  23, 27, 39, 41, 43, 44,
  47, 52, 53, 55, 59, 60,
  64, 67, 82, 93, 99, 104,
  124, 230, 258, 261, 264,
  266
natural, xviii, 10, 19, 21,
  22, 24, 25, 27, 38, 49,
  68, 69, 71, 73, 107, 114,
  117, 130, 144, 164, 165,
  183, 185, 214, 225, 243,
  251, 252, 263
oral routes (pills), 28
osteoporosis/bones, xiv, 8,
  19, 20, 22, 31, 39, 42,
  43, 54, 55, 59, 67, 74,
  77, 121, 162, 229, 230,
  251, 262, 267
ovary/ovary removal
  (oophorectomy), 33, 46,
  53
patches, xviii, xix, 15, 28,
  33, 34, 51, 76, 185
pellets, x, xix, 16, 21, 34,
  35, 36, 37, 38, 39, 40,
  41, 42, 43, 44, 45, 46,
  48, 51, 52, 53, 54, 55,

56, 57, 59, 61, 66, 72,
  76, 78, 94, 106
perimenopause, 39, 49
postmenopause/menopaus
  e, ix, xviii, xix, xxi, xxii,
  15, 16, 17, 18, 20, 22,
  23, 27, 39, 41, 43, 44,
  47, 52, 53, 55, 59, 60,
  64, 67, 82, 93, 99, 104,
  124, 230, 258, 261, 264,
  266
premenopausal estrogen
  level/ratios, 37, 41, 70
sexual response, 52
shots, xx, 50, 109
side effects, x, xi, xviii, 4,
  9, 16, 21, 22, 44, 61, 64,
  77, 78, 90, 106, 108,
  140, 141, 185, 193
sublinguals, 28, 43, 75,
  76, 239
testosterone, x, xi, xx, xxii,
  6, 9, 16, 17, 20, 23, 26,
  28, 34, 35, 36, 38, 41,
  42, 43, 44, 45, 46, 47,
  50, 52, 54, 56, 58, 60,
  61, 62, 63, 64, 65, 66,
  67, 68, 69, 70, 71, 72,
  73, 74, 75, 76, 77, 78,
  80, 91, 106, 183, 193,
  194, 216, 222, 226, 227,
  228, 264, 265, 266, 267
vaginal, 15, 18, 39, 55, 63,
  236
Human Growth Hormone
  (HGH), xii, 105
Hypertension, xiv, 3, 4, 18,
  22, 59, 77, 78, 82, 97, 99,

159, 202, 211, 213, 224, 228, 261, 269
Hypothyroidism, xi, xii, xxii, 81, 82, 83, 91, 93, 94, 95, 96, 97, 98, 99, 100, 101, 102, 103, 104, 123, 237, 267
  diagnosis, xii, 99, 104
  symptoms, xxii, 100, 101
  treatment, 101
Infections, 3, 5, 18, 136, 137, 147, 150, 151, 236
Inflammations, xii, xvii, xxiii, 5, 10, 11, 26, 27, 28, 58, 69, 79, 80, 86, 91, 116, 120, 126, 127, 128, 129, 130, 131, 134, 138, 139, 140, 145, 147, 158, 174, 182, 195, 212, 213, 214, 215, 216, 217, 219, 222, 224, 225, 226, 227, 228
Infrared sauna, 172, 173
Insomnia, xvii, 18, 26, 39, 40, 57, 66, 67, 73, 77, 79, 82, 83, 91, 122, 177, 191, 194, 251
Insulin, xiv, 8, 20, 23, 25, 34, 46, 58, 73, 81, 86, 99, 100, 106, 109, 115, 122, 124, 125, 126, 127, 128, 131, 134, 214, 215, 216, 223, 224, 225, 226, 251, 269
Intercourse, painful, 15
Interstitial cystitis, 47, 49
Iodine, 97, 100, 102, 123
irritable bowel syndrome, 80, 83, 91, 138, 177, 219

Kidneys, 4, 79, 109, 128, 135, 154, 157, 165, 170, 220, 230, 236
Laboratory, 60, 108, 129, 141
LDL, 213
Lead, 161, 162
Leaky gut syndrome, xxii, 83, 177
Libido, xvii, xx, xxiii, 15, 16, 20, 22, 31, 34, 39, 41, 44, 45, 54, 57, 63, 65, 66, 73, 74, 77, 78, 94, 96, 98, 191, 193
Lipids, 34
lipoproteins, 213
  high-density lipoproteins, 213
  low-density lipoproteins, 213
liver, 4, 27, 28, 34, 43, 58, 68, 75, 76, 89, 109, 118, 119, 120, 121, 122, 123, 124, 135, 140, 154, 157, 158, 160, 161, 165, 166, 167, 168, 169, 174, 177, 214, 220, 221, 223, 224, 226, 236
low blood pressure (see blood pressure), 86
Low-density lipoproteins (LDL), 213
lymphatic system, 165, 170
Magnesium, 10, 58, 85, 89, 91, 102, 121, 122, 138, 144, 160, 161, 168, 169, 216, 225, 231, 239, 269
Medicine, future of, 105

Meditation, xiii, xxiii, 85, 87, 196, 197, 203, 221, 253
  ancient arts, 203
Melatonin, 9, 23, 26, 58, 85, 191, 195, 222, 228, 239, 264
Memory, xiv, xvii, xviii, 18, 25, 27, 31, 39, 52, 54, 59, 73, 74, 77, 78, 81, 83, 90, 106, 138, 147, 155, 158, 189, 190, 191, 192, 193, 197, 226, 229, 235, 250, 251, 267
Men, xx, xxii, 16, 20, 28, 46, 56, 65, 66, 68, 69, 70, 73, 74, 75, 76, 77, 78, 94, 96, 106, 193, 194, 211, 216, 218, 229, 237, 265, 266, 267, 268
  Aging, xi, 70, 74
  bio-identical hormone replacement, 44, 59, 66, 237
  testosterone, x, xi, xx, xxii, 6, 9, 16, 17, 20, 23, 26, 28, 34, 35, 36, 38, 41, 42, 43, 44, 45, 46, 47, 50, 52, 54, 56, 58, 60, 61, 62, 63, 64, 65, 66, 67, 68, 69, 70, 71, 72, 73, 74, 75, 76, 77, 78, 80, 91, 106, 183, 193, 194, 216, 222, 226, 227, 228, 264, 265, 266, 267
Menopause/postmenopause, ix, xviii, xix, xxi, xxii, 15, 16, 17, 18, 20, 22, 23, 27, 39, 41, 43, 44, 47, 52, 53, 55, 59, 60, 64, 67, 82, 93,

99, 104, 124, 230, 258, 261, 264, 266
Mercury, xx, xxii, 118, 123, 149, 150, 151, 157, 158, 159, 160, 161, 162, 163, 164, 176, 177, 249, 268
  chelation, 150, 161, 162
  diagnosis, 159
  source, 158
  treatment, 160
Metabolism, 22, 65, 81, 88, 96, 125, 161, 193, 226, 262
  Carbohydrate, 20
  first-pass, 27
  glucose/blood sugar, 34, 122
  hormone, 27
Methylation, 166, 168, 214
Mind-Body connection, xiii, 187
  Brain, 188
  meditation, 196
  self-esteem, xiii, 198
Mitochondria, 10, 89, 95, 122, 157, 216, 229
Neurodegenerative diseases, xxiii, 109, 152, 177, 227
Neuroendocrine, ix, xiii, 8, 190, 194, 228
  Theory, ix, xxii, 7, 8, 17, 219
Neurotransmitter, 19, 82, 190, 191, 192, 193, 229
Nitric oxide, 213
Nutrition, xii, xiv, xxiii, 3, 5, 12, 39, 58, 102, 107, 113, 126, 133, 145, 172, 176,

183, 186, 194, 213, 222, 242

food allergies, xx, 97, 100, 128, 133, 136, 142, 143, 145, 147

Obesity, xiv, 12, 68, 99, 136, 202, 213, 223, 228, 251, 266, 269

Olive oil, 116, 119, 143, 169, 242, 244, 245

Omega 3 fatty acid, 116, 118, 127, 129, 174, 195, 217, 222, 227, 228, 249

Organic food, 127

Organochlorides, pesticides, 153

Organophosphates, 155

Osteoarthritis, 51

Osteopenia, xiv, 19, 54, 55, 77, 229, 230

Osteoporosis/bones, xiv, 8, 19, 20, 22, 31, 39, 42, 43, 54, 55, 59, 67, 74, 77, 121, 162, 229, 230, 251, 262, 267

Oxidative stress, 10, 11, 158, 162, 212

Painful intercourse, 22, 39, 236

Pancreatic enzyme, 134

Patches, xviii, xix, 15, 28, 33, 34, 51, 76, 185
  Estrogens, 28
  testosterone, 28

PCB (polychlorinated biphenols), 154

Pellets (hormone), xix, 16, 33, 34, 51, 54, 61, 94, 149
  estrogen, 43, 106

testosterone, xx, 74

Periods, 18, 60, 96, 98, 103

Pesticides, 57, 69, 97, 102, 113, 126, 127, 152, 153, 155, 163, 164, 165, 166, 176, 220, 252, 267

Phosphatidylserine, 229

Physiological, 26, 30, 34, 43, 64, 76, 77, 78, 90, 106, 264

Pituitary gland, 8, 36, 60, 98, 99, 105, 188, 189

Plastics/plasricizers, 57, 69, 98, 102, 155, 156, 157, 166, 220

PMS, x, 19, 62, 119, 191, 194, 202

Potassium, 80, 81, 123, 124, 138, 216

Probiotics, 58, 136, 142, 144, 145, 147, 168, 171, 249

Progesterone, xviii, 9, 15, 16, 17, 19, 20, 21, 23, 24, 25, 26, 28, 38, 41, 43, 49, 50, 56, 58, 60, 61, 63, 80, 91, 192, 193, 194, 222, 261, 263, 264

Progestin, 15, 25, 263

Prostaglandins, 116, 139

Prostate cancer, xxiii, 56, 68, 69, 77, 151, 153, 156, 217, 218, 265

Prostate gland, 69

Prostate hypertrophy, 68, 69, 77

Protein, 46, 68, 73, 86, 105, 115, 118, 119, 127, 128, 129, 134, 166, 174, 195, 214

Saliva test, 40, 84
Saturated fat, 116, 117, 128
Sauna, 172, 173
Saw palmetto, 69, 78
Sea vegetables, 128
Selenium, 58, 78, 89, 91,
    102, 122, 123, 160, 161,
    167, 216, 222, 225
Serotonin, 18, 85, 190, 191,
    192, 193, 195, 239
Sex drive/libido, 45, 54, 55,
    66, 83, 96, 98
Sex hormone binding
    globulin (SBGH), 60, 67
Sex hormones/steroids, xxi,
    xxii, 16, 18, 59, 60, 64, 82,
    101, 103, 106, 156, 236
Silent spring, 153
Skin, xiii, 19, 163, 179, 181,
    182, 183, 184, 185, 226,
    234
Sleep, xiv, 84, 235, 237, 238,
    239
Spirit/Mind-body
    connection, xii, 111
    subconscious, power of,
        203
Stem Cells, 107, 108, 109
    Hgh, 105
    regenerative medicine,
        109
    research, 107, 109
    treatments, xii, 105, 107
Stress, xi, xiv, xvii, xxi, xxii,
    xxiii, 3, 4, 5, 10, 12, 26,
    37, 56, 58, 59, 79, 80, 82,
    83, 84, 86, 87, 90, 91, 100,
    103, 109, 186, 193, 194,
    213, 216, 221, 226, 227,
    228, 237, 239, 240, 241,
    242, 251, 259
Adrenal, 60, 81, 82
    chronic, xx, xxi, 47, 217
    oxidative, ix, 9, 10, 11,
        158, 162, 212
    reduction, 58, 91, 103,
        186, 194, 216, 221, 226,
        228
Stroke, xiv, 159, 211
Sublingual (hormones), 28,
    43, 75, 76, 239
Supplements, xi, 58, 88, 89,
    195, 216, 222, 225, 239,
    249
    Detoxification, 226
    diabetes, 224
Synthetic hormones, 20, 21,
    33, 37
T3 (triiodothyronine), 23, 60,
    81, 100, 101, 102, 103,
    104
T4 (thyroxine), 60, 81, 100,
    101, 102, 103, 104
Telomeres, ix, 7
Testosterone Deficiency, 63,
    71, 78
Testosterone receptor, 70
Testosterone/androgen
    abdominal fat, 68, 73
    adrenal glands, xxi, xxii,
        9, 17, 46, 47, 60, 79, 80,
        81, 82, 84, 85, 88, 89,
        90, 91, 94, 103, 189, 192
    aging, xi, 70, 74
    Alzheimer's disease, 73
    blood pressure, 77
    bones/osteoporosis, xi, 74
    brain, 70

breast cancer, 77
cardiovascular disease, x, 70
cholesterol, 70
creams, 75
deficiency, x, 44, 63, 65, 67, 71, 78
dementia, 70
depression, x, 69
diagnosis, iv, 45, 60, 83, 91, 95, 104, 137, 177, 229
estrogen, x, 68
fatigue, 41
hair, 67
insulin/diabetes, x, 71
jointpain, 39, 67, 99, 147, 176, 235
lab/test levels, 66, 70, 71, 73, 77, 78
libido, 41
memory, 22, 67, 73, 82, 98, 191
migraines, 19, 41, 42, 54, 63, 177, 191
muscles, 70
oral/pills, 75
ovary/ovaries, 82
patches, 28
pellets, 42
prostate, x, 68
PSA, 76
replacements, 73
shots, 76
skin, xiii, xviii, 7, 15, 16, 19, 28, 29, 30, 35, 37, 40, 51, 54, 55, 63, 64, 66, 75, 76, 98, 99, 103, 106, 107, 119, 120, 121,
123, 125, 133, 142, 145, 147, 157, 163, 164, 179, 180, 181, 182, 183, 184, 185, 186, 218, 220, 223, 226, 234
sleep/insomnia, 73
sublingual, 75
weight, xii, xvii, xxii, xxiii, 3, 4, 6, 7, 15, 16, 22, 34, 39, 40, 54, 66, 67, 71, 72, 73, 77, 81, 82, 93, 94, 98, 103, 115, 127, 128, 131, 137, 145, 170, 215, 221, 225, 226, 231, 235, 250, 252, 253
Thyroid gland thyroid stimulating hormone, 8, 36, 59, 98, 99
Thyroid hormone, 6, 8, 23, 31, 58, 60, 81, 93, 94, 95, 96, 97, 98, 101, 102, 103, 104, 123, 193, 194, 226, 227
Thyroxine, 100, 267
Toxic avoidance, 102, 177
Toxins/toxic, xii, xiii, xiv, 5, 79, 102, 145, 149, 153, 164, 170, 177, 224, 236, 252
Trace minerals, 89
Trans fats, 86
triiodothyronine, 100
TSH (see thyroid stimulating hormone), 8, 60, 98, 99, 100
Tumors
fibroids, 62
Turmeric, 127, 128, 131, 143, 148, 174, 250

Ultrasound, 61, 70, 100, 218, 220
Ultraviolet rays, 179
Urinary tract, bladder/interstitial cystitis, 47
Uterus/uterine, 18, 19, 33, 38, 49, 61, 62, 202
Vagina/vaginal, 15, 18, 39, 55, 63, 236
dryness, 15, 18, 63
Vasodilator/vasodilation, 216
Vegetables, 10, 86, 88, 89, 113, 114, 115, 119, 120, 121, 122, 124, 125, 127, 128, 129, 130, 131, 143, 146, 163, 164, 169, 172, 173, 215, 221, 225, 227, 231, 243, 244, 247, 254
Vitamin A, 119, 135, 166, 167, 183, 231
Vitamin B complex, 229
Vitamin B1, 119, 144
Vitamin B2, 119, 144
Vitamin B3, 166
Vitamin B6, 89, 166, 214, 216
Vitamin C, 88, 89, 120, 162, 167, 174, 216, 221, 222, 250
Vitamin D, 121, 231

Vitamin E, 88, 89, 120, 121, 122, 167, 183, 185, 214, 216, 222
Vitamin K, 135
Vitamins, 89, 113, 119, 120
Water, 10, 11, 37, 47, 61, 63, 87, 97, 98, 102, 104, 119, 124, 125, 126, 127, 130, 131, 135, 143, 152, 154, 156, 157, 163, 164, 168, 169, 170, 171, 172, 173, 174, 177, 180, 181, 182, 185, 221, 225, 231, 238, 243, 244, 245, 246, 247, 249, 255, 267, 269
drinking, 98, 126
Extracellular, 126
intracellular, 125, 126
polluted, 157
retention, 61, 63, 126, 181
Weight gain, xvii, xxiii, 39, 40, 54, 66, 67, 77, 81, 82, 98, 115, 145, 226, 235
Women's Health Initiative, 23, 31, 261, 262
Xenohormones, 57, 68, 127, 220
Zinc, 58, 68, 69, 78, 89, 91, 102, 123, 137, 160, 161, 167, 182, 225, 231